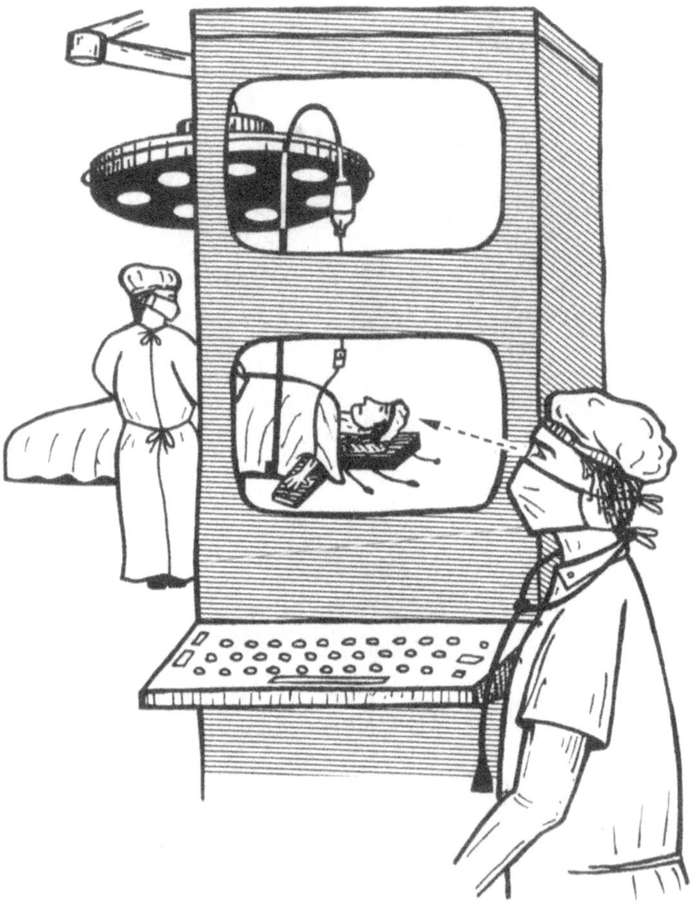

Annejet P. Meijler

Automation in Anesthesia – A Relief?

A Systematic Approach to Computers in Patient Monitoring

Foreword by J. E. W. Beneken

With 69 Figures and 22 Tables

Springer-Verlag
Berlin Heidelberg New York
London Paris Tokyo

Dr. Annejet P. Meijler
University of Technology, Den Dolech 2
P.O. Box 513, NL-5600 MB Eindhoven

ISBN-13:978-3-540-18204-7 e-ISBN-13:978-3-642-72913-3
DOI: 10.1007/978-3-642-72913-3

Library of Congress Cataloging-in-Publication Data
Meijler, A.P. (Annejet P.), 1954- . Automation in anesthesia.
Bibliography: p. Includes index. 1. Anesthesia - Data processing. 2. Patient monitoring - Data processing. 3. Microcomputers. I. Title. [DNLM: 1. Anesthesia. 2. Monitoring, Physiologic - methods. 3. Signal Processing, Computer-Assisted. WO 200 M512a]
RD80.95.M45 1987 617'.96'0285 87-24332

2119/3140-543210

To Whom I Love

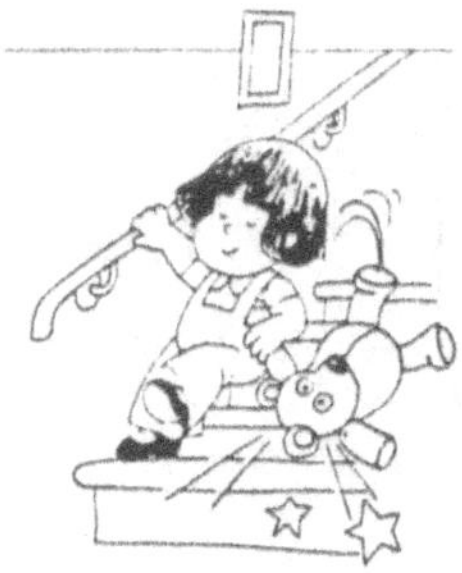

It is as far as the bear knows,
the *only* way of coming downstairs . . . . .
but sometimes he *feels,*
there is really *another way* . . . . .
if only he could *stop* bumping
for a moment and *think* of it!!

(From: A. A. Milne, Winnie-the-Pooh)

Foreword

Anesthesia is a fascinating area because it deals with the patient as a whole. The anesthesiologist takes full responsibility for the patient and his physiological well-being during a period which may become live-threatening if no proper surveillance were available. This is the essence of the complexity of anesthesia. The providing of the conditions for the surgeons to operate on the patient is, although originally the primary goal, probably no longer the most difficult aspect.

The anesthesiologist is faced with a growing number of variables he needs to monitor. Not only the measurements are of his concern, the interpretation of the individual signals and, even more, the assessment of the (cor)relation between the signals and their variations require his full attention.

Many attempts have been made to place the individual instruments together which resulted in ergonomically better situations. The advent of multichannel displays, some making use of as many colors as possible, raised questions about the optimal display: what is optimal, is that true for all situations, can we judge that objectively, how important is the subjective feeling of the user?

These questions are too general to permit a direct answer. With this study we tried to answer many of these questions for a particular case, cardioanesthesia, because we felt that this was probably the most complex situation and that many of the results could be applied in less complex patient monitoring situations.

This book gives a description of the development and function of a data acquisition and display system on the basis of a thorough problem analysis. It is, however, even more important that the methodology that is developed is germane to many monitoring situations, now and in the future.

Eindhoven, July 1987

Jan E. W. Beneken
Professor of
Medical Electrical Engineering

Preface

The work reported in this book, a revised version of my Ph. D. thesis, was carried out within the Division of Medical Electrical Engineering (head: Prof. J. E. W. Beneken) from the Eindhoven University of Technology and at the Department of Anesthesiology (head: Prof. Joh. Spierdijk) of the University Hospital Leyden. The project was supported in part by the Netherlands Technology Foundation (STW) and Honeywell Medical Electronics B. V. (currently PPG Hellige).

Nowadays most research is not performed by one single person. This is especially true for the multi-disciplinary subject described in this book, in which we worked on the boundary between human engineering and medical engineering. As a consequence I am indebted to a great many people.

In the first place I would like to thank my first promotor, Professor J. E. W. Beneken. He was the master-mind behind the servo-anesthesia project of which the research in this book is a part. In spite of the fact that his clinic was invaded by technicians, my second promotor, Professor Joh. Spierdijk, gave all possible support for the practical realization of the tests performed in the ORs. I am very grateful to my friends and teachers from the Medical Physics Lab in Amsterdam: Dr. T. J. T. P. van den Berg and Professor L. H. van der Tweel for the stimulating discussions and the co-editing of this work.

Without the contribution made by my colleagues H. van Kessel and J. Blom this work could not have been realized. An essential contribution in the development and clinical testing of the computerized monitoring system DADS came from the physicians A. Nandorff, P. Hennis, R. Nelissen, J. R. de Jong and H. van Wezel. P. Damman gave his immeasurable support in the form of text editing and programming. J. Onink was very patient with my continuous updating of his professionally made figures. Furthermore, I want to express my thanks to everybody, both in the University Hospital of Leyden and at the Eindhoven University of Technology, who gave their invaluable support to this project.

My parents gave me the education and love which are fundamental to everything. Kees, I could not have managed without your unwavering support and your trust both in me and in the completion of this work.

Eindhoven, July 1987 Annejet P. Meijler

Contents

Abbreviations

N. B. Abbreviations which are listed elsewhere are not included.

ACT	Activated Clotting Time
AIS	Anesthesia Information System
ASA	American Society of Anesthesiologists
AV	Surface area outside zone around running average of signal
C	Free comment command of DADS
CI	Cardiac Index
CO	Cardiac Output
CO_2	Carbon Dioxide
CPB	Cardiopulmonary Bypass
CRT	Color Ray Tube
CVP	Central Venous Pressure
DADS	Data Acquisition and Display System
ECG	Electrocardiogram
FAFR	Fatal Accident Frequency Rate
FLOW	Flowchart
HIS	Histogram
HR	Heart-Rate
ICU	Intensive Care Unit
L rel	Relative Luminance
LED	Light Emitting Diode
LVEDP	Left Ventricular End Diastolic Pressure
M	Surface area outside zone around mathematical mean of signal
MAP	Mean Arterial Pressure
MCVP	Mean Central Venous Pressure
MIVOL	Minute Volume
N	Surface area outside zone around normal value of signal
NTG	Nitroglycerin (vasodilator)
N_2O	Nitrous Oxide

O_2	Oxygen
OK	"Operatie Kamer"
OR	Operating Room
PAP	Pulmonary Arterial Pressure
PART	Arterial Pressure
PAWP	Pulmonary Arterial Wedge Pressure
PDIA	Diastolic Arterial Pressure
PO_2	Partial Oxygen Tension
PCO_2	Partial Carbon Dioxide Tension
PRMX	Maximal Respiratory Pressure
PSYS	Systolic Arterial Pressure
Q	Free comment command containing quantitative information
RRATE	Respiratory Rate
SNP	Sodium Nitroprusside (vasodilator)
SPSS	Statistical Package for the Social Sciences
SVR	Systemic Vascular Resistance
VENT	Ventilation signals

1 General Introduction

1.1 Introduction and Survey

Utilizing tools in order to accomplish tasks beyond the limit of human performance is inherent to man. As early as 400,000 years ago, homo sapiens used tools made of stone to club down elephants (Fig. 1.1) (Johanson and Edey 1981). This aspect of human behavior has not changed since. At present we are living in an era in which automation is used to expand our abilities.

According to Toffler (1980): "computers [are], linked to banks, stores, government offices, to neighbor's homes and to the workplace, destined to reshape not only business, from production to retailing, but the very nature of work and, indeed, even the structure of the family."

This book discusses one aspect of automation: its possibilities and the justification of its use in (cardio)anesthesia. Specifically: the evaluation of an automated data acquisition and display system (DADS) for patient monitoring will be treated. A generally applicable evaluation method was composed. Its execution required the consideration of the usual procedures at and around cardioanesthesia from different viewpoints. The objective of the evaluation was to detect over a broad range the possible weak spots in the work situation of the cardioanesthesiol-

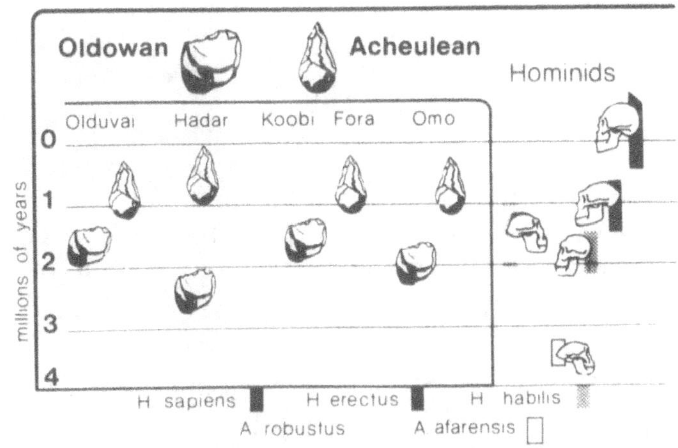

Fig. 1.1 From the concurrency in findings of tools and bones, according to site and age, it was deduced that tools of this kind must be an invention of homo and that homo habilis may turn out to be 2.5 millions of years old. (From Johanson and Edey 1981).

ogist and to determine whether these can be improved by means of extensions to DADS or by the application of other possibilities. That improvements in anesthesia, in spite of its degree of perfection, are still possible can be illustrated by means of the so-called FAFR values for different occupations. FAFR is short for Fatal Accident Frequency Rate. This is the number of fatal accidents per 100,000,000 hours spent in a specific situation. For the year 1980 Zelders (1986) quoted from various sources the following FAFR values (which apply to the Netherlands unless stated otherwise):

Pregnancy	1
Railroad traffic	5
Car traffic	6
Agriculture	10
Traffic (general)	50
Construction	67
Air traffic (international)	100
Anesthesia	4000

Thus, in comparison with other common activities, the risk in being under anesthesia, iatrogenic causes (as far as possible) excluded, is considerable. To obtain an impression of the number of fatalities per year, these numbers must be corrected for the number of hours spent in a specific situation. For instance, the number of fatalities in traffic is about 2000 per year while in anesthesia this is (estimated at) only 70 per year. The reason for this is that the number of hours spent in traffic is 2500 times higher than the time spent on the operating table. But still the fatalities in anesthesia are deemed to be of public importance: according to an estimation by Spierdijk (priv. comm. 1985) $1.2 \cdot 10^6$ anesthetic procedures are performed each year in the Netherlands. This means that on the average the Dutchman will have to undergo anesthesia once every 10 years.

The FAFR, however, is only a measure for the tip of the iceberg, namely the fatalities. In traffic for instance, the number of injured persons is about 55000 per year.

In aviation a special technique has been developed which in addition to fatal accidents, systematically uses all near accidents to obtain information which can be used for preventive measures.

In anesthesia these so-called "critical incidents" are also becoming of increasing importance in relation to prevention. Cooper et al. (1978) gave the following definition for a critical incident in anesthesia:

> "A mishap was labeled a critical incident when it was clearly an occurrence that could have led (if not discovered and corrected in time) or did lead to an undesirable outcome, ranging from increased length of hospital stay to death or permanent disability."

However, as we will see later, the so-called critical incident technique is not yet at an adequate stage to trace the mishaps with satisfactory accuracy.

Until now, most investigators have attempted to identify problem areas directly related to the tasks of the anesthesiologist. These include monitoring, controlling and data logging. A well-known problem in data logging was quantified by Zol-

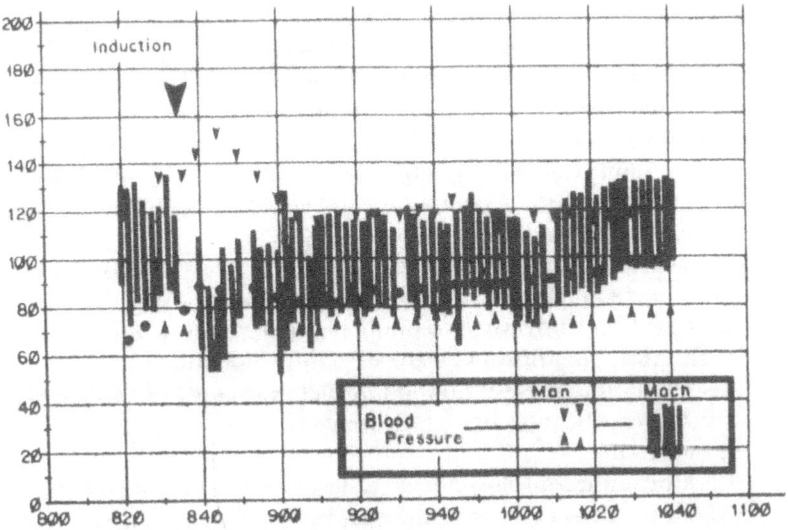

Fig. 1.2 There are often considerable discrepancies between values as registered by an automatic data logger and values on the handwritten anesthesia record, such as shown here after induction of anesthesia. (From Zollinger et al. (1977), by permission of Academic Press).

linger et al. (1977). From the 100 cases where a drop in blood pressure was recorded by an automatic data logger, 40 went unrecorded on the handwritten anesthesia record (Fig. 1.2). Paget et al. (1981) explain that human vigilance and therewith the quality of monitoring decreases after 10 minutes. Smith (1983) showed that when a correct model can be realized the corresponding control task is performed better by a machine. In this context Beneken et al. (1974) tried to model halothane controlled anesthesia. They noticed, however, that many types of measurement were not sufficiently accurate to be able to control the physiological signals. In addition, they noticed a few other problems such as decentralized data presentation and a low level of data processing as factors which inhibit fast decision making for the anesthesiologists.

These problems led to our servoanesthesia project, designed to assess the degree to which automation in anesthesia is useful. In the extreme, the project is directed toward a closed-loop anesthesia delivery station comparable to the automatic pilot in aviation: not a system designed to dispense with the anesthesiologist but a system tailored to take over time-consuming, tedious and programmable tasks. As a starting point, we developed DADS for centralized measuring and surveyable information presentation. During its development the need for a systematic evaluation (test and improvement phase) was recognized. In principle, the system has been designed to be applicable during any type of surgical procedure. However, in the systematic evaluation of the system, as treated in this book, we have restricted ourselves to one type of procedure which puts high demands on the quality of monitoring: namely the cardioanesthetic procedure.

The need for the evaluation of DADS arose, amongst other things, because the anesthesiologists came up with many suggestions regarding extensions and improvements to DADS. A guide to priority setting was deemed necessary and the assignment was to expand this to the setting up of a more organized design protocol for comparable systems. Another major issue was that if experiences with such a system are positive this does not automatically imply that patient care is measurably improved. Just as with the introduction of a new pharmacon, one would like to show an improvement in patient care to justify yet another piece of equipment in the operating room. Therefore, we included experiments to test the impact of DADS on the course of anesthesia.

Summarizing: in the evaluation, attention has been given to the detection of possible new requirements for DADS on different levels:

- the signal level: to provide optimal support in decision making it is essential that clinically significant signal behavior is identified.
- the organizational level: to minimize the existence of factors which may lead to critical incidents, the work (environment) of the (cardio)anesthesiologist has to be improved.
- the critical incident level: direct studies into critical incidents are likely to provide us with clear clues as to the aspects in which automation may be most useful.

In Section 1.2 we will mention some of the historical developments which have led to such a complex situation in the operating room that the application of automation seems necessary.

Following this introduction, Chapter 2 will present in detail the problems which underly the topic of this book, and is dedicated to a description of the task of the anesthesiologist in the operating room. The following matters will be treated: a general impression of anesthetic management, the subtasks and workload of the anesthesiologist, and the layout of the operating room. Various problems will be discussed, where possible, suggestions for improvement will be given and some will be elaborated upon in subsequent chapters.

In Chapter 3 (on materials) those aspects of DADS will be described which are of importance for the user and the evaluation of DADS. This means that a description of the fundamental software and hardware will not be included; for this we refer to the several master theses which have been written on these subjects: Hengst en Krämer (1980), van Kessel (1981), te Dorsthorst (1982), Hees (1983), van de Lavoir (1983), Heesbeen (1984), Coolegem (1984). It must be realized that in this book DADS is, in fact, both the subject of the investigation, namely the system to be evaluated, and the measuring instrument: the system for collecting the data which will be used to learn more about decision making by the anesthesiologist.

Chapter 4 (on methods) describes the evaluation method as composed and applied in this book. It starts with a review of evaluation methods as applied by others on comparable systems. Though many elements have been used in these methods, they have mostly been incomplete from the human engineering point of view. To our knowledge there is no systematic basic method from which these elements have been carefully selected. Therefore we composed a general evaluation method which will be presented against the background of human engineering guidelines. Subsequently, the evaluation method as applicable to DADS will be described; it is a selection of the possible tests and techniques as mentioned in the general evaluation method.

The clinical evaluation is treated in Chapter 5. It includes the experiments which were carried out in order to test the performance of DADS. Two tests will be described. The first test was developed to check the clinical significance of the alarms generated by an objective algorithm in DADS.

In the second test the deviation of physiological signals from their normal zones is used as the criterion to test whether monitoring by DADS has a measurable influence on signal behavior and therewith possibly on patient care.

Chapter 6 details some major improvements and changes in the ergonomics (layout, man-machine interaction, data presentation) of DADS. Many new requirements for DADS were collected during course of the evaluation. Small improvements and suggestions are discussed where relevant in the various chapters and have been implemented when possible. The improvements to be described in Chapter 6 have not been developed and tested in vivo, but have been used by the industry as the instigation for a commercially integrated workstation (Zegers-de Beyl 1985), and they resulted for us in the design of a "maxi-DADS": an integrated workstation for research applications.

Chapter 7 discusses another improvement to DADS. It describes the major extension effected to DADS: the automated anesthesia record. A separate evaluation, which was performed by means of a brief questionnaire to determine the satisfaction of the users with the record, is also treated.

Chapter 8 contains recommendations. When automation is applied in the operating room, a primary goal should be to decrease critical incidents; therefore we present a literature study regarding critical incidents in anesthesia. It will be shown that, though DADS may avert some of the factors associated with critical incidents, it is not (yet) directly designed for the prevention of critical incidents. Recommendations for adapting systems like DADS in order to prevent some critical incidents are given.

1.2 Historical Developments in Monitoring

Through the ages it has been the task of the physician to watch and observe the patient with the specific purpose (=monitoring) of making a diagnosis and/or performing a therapeutic action. Nowadays the task of "monitoring" is often mentioned in one breath with the monitoring equipment. Therefore it is not clear whether the medical conception of monitoring does or does not include the observation of the clinical signs without an aid. This also follows from the different definitions of monitoring. Spierdijk and Nandorff (1974) define monitoring as "the continuous visualization of specific measured phenomena, which can be performed in either an analog (graphic) or digital (numerical) fashion". Collins (1981) defines monitoring as "the repetitive performance of observations and measurements intended to detect a specific event, to follow the clinical course, or to evaluate therapeutic response". The second definition is broader than the first and includes observation of both the clinical signs and the phenomena as presented by additional measuring equipment. Ream (1982, p139) even includes the control task in his definition of monitoring. According to de Lange (1985) there is no difference between monitoring with and without equipment: the transducers which enable man to observe the state of the patient more clearly are just extensions of the senses. Thus, directly observable clinical signs and parameters which can only be (correctly) observed by means of "transducers" must both be included in the monitoring. However, it should be noted that the specific monitoring equipment is not the only equipment which has to be monitored by the anesthesiologist, whose main commission during surgery is to bring the patient into and maintain a state which enables the execution of a surgical procedure and secures the vital functions of the patient.

In order to realize this, additional equipment is required: during cardiac surgical procedures indispensable equipment includes a ventilator and, also of major importance, a cardiopulmonary bypass (CPB) apparatus. The latter is essential for taking over the pumping function of the heart and the oxygenation by the lung during periods when the activity of the heart is stopped to enable the surgeons to operate on the heart itself.

Pieces of equipment like this present the anesthesiologist with additional sets of parameters to be monitored and/or adjusted. Summarizing, the monitoring task of the anesthesiologist regards parameters from:

S- Directly observable clinical signs (around 12; see pp. 12-13)
A- The anesthesia delivery machine
V- The ventilator (A and V are coupled or integrated for cardiac procedures)
H- The hemodynamic monitoring equipment including temperatures
B- The cardiopulmonary bypass apparatus (monitored and controlled by pump technicians but in concert with the anesthesiologist)
G- Blood gas and electrolyte values as determined outside the operating room
I- Intravenous infusions
M- Administered medications
F- Fluid balance (blood,plasma,drip infusion in, soaked bandages,blood,urinary out)
R- Recording devices

In each of these categories, advanced knowledge and technology are required to enable monitoring during cardiac anesthesia. The breakthrough to cardiac surgery was the realization by Gibbon (1954) of the CPB apparatus, with which he performed the first successful cardiac surgical procedure. Years later, in 1969, the first aortocoronary bypass operation in the Netherlands was reported (Laird-Meeter 1983). At present, around 7500 bypass operations per year are performed in the Netherlands under the care of anesthesiologists specially trained for cardiac cases.

Numerous advances in science had to be made, however, before the breakthrough to cardiac surgery could take place (Wood 1978). Some of them are marked in Fig. 1.3, in which time lines for some of the categories included in monitoring are given. One essential milestone was that, in the middle of the 19th century, the agents ether, nitrous oxide and chloroform were introduced to induce anesthesia. From this point modern anesthesiology evolved and allowed an enormous expansion in surgery because at last painless treatment was possible. A comprehensive overview of the developments in anesthesiology is given by Lee and

Atkinson (1973). The discovery of anesthetics meant only the start of an era: an era in which the ventilator, developing since the 18th century, grew into a sophisticated tool enabling anesthesiology to become an independent specialty in the US and the western European countries circa 1945.

Comroe and Dripps (1976) performed an impressively thorough analysis of the scientific research which led to cardiac surgery. After studying 4000 articles they

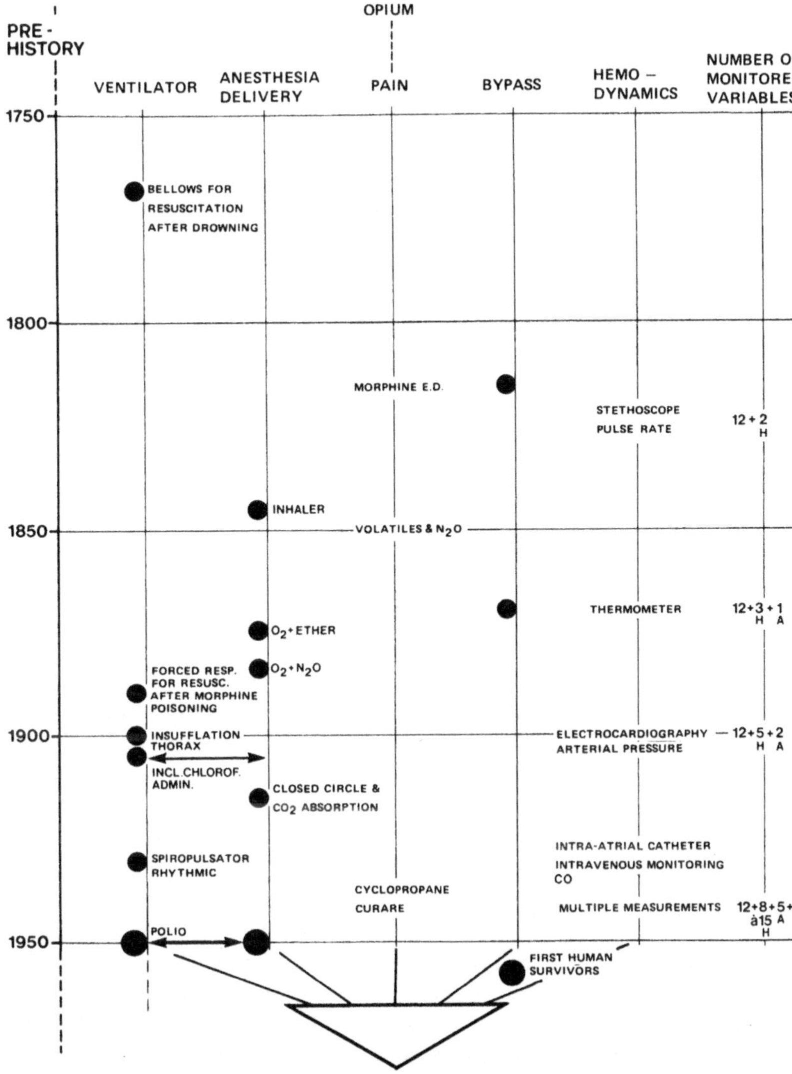

Fig. 1.3 Important steps in the development on specific subjects are marked in several time lines. Most of the time, developments took place independently. Together they enable cardiac surgery, but at the same time result in a steady increase of the variables which have to be monitored. In the time line on the right the number of variables to be monitored and their origin are indicated: clinical signs (S), anesthesia delivery machine (A), hemodynamic monitoring equipment (H), etc. (see p. 6).

showed that 40% of the research which ultimately enabled cardiac surgery had not been clinically oriented at the time of the research. Knowledge was obtained for its own sake, and was not directed toward cardiac surgery. Comroe (1978), in *Retroscope*, gives many interesting examples regarding the causes of major developments: there were often very different motivations for their initiation. For instance the ventilator was initiated to resuscitate people after near drowning (Kaplan 1983) and after morphine poisoning (Comroe 1978). Moreover, further development of the different devices was, in most cases, independent. Apart from technical barriers, this precluded right from the start any notions regarding integration or attuning of the equipment.

Yet there have been periods of exchange between the lines of development. At the start of the 20th century attempts were made to perform surgical procedures in the thorax, and this required both the administration of anesthetics and the prevention of lung collapse. A system for both insufflation and the administration of chloroform was applied (Kaplan 1983), but this did not result in further combined development.

In Fig. 1.3, the right-hand line gives the number of directly observable clinical signs such as perspiration and pupil size, which remains constant (about 12) over the years. In addition to these, the number of indirect signals grows consistently. The new hemodynamic parameters which can be monitored and also, and not negligibly, the data presented by the ventilation and anesthesia delivery systems form part of this. At first, the anesthesiologist observed only the supply of volatiles in an inhaler. However, from the beginning of the 20th century parameters such as pressures and flows in delivery systems are included and, later still, ventilation pressures, flows, frequency, volume and cycle parameters.

This implies that, at the time cardiac surgery became reality, the anesthesiologist had if he could, to monitor about 30 variables. In spite of the advances along all lines of development following this breakthrough, no essential changes took place with respect to the number and diversity of variables to be monitored. Therefore it is not surprising that, when we consider the current state of the art in the operating room, the impression is that the various devices are often very sophisticated but that the total layout is diverse and unintegrated.

Fig. 1.4 is an illustration of an arrangement of equipment: an operating room for cardiac surgery in the University Hospital of Leyden, where most of the investigations to be described in this book were performed. The scattered presentation of the information can be seen clearly. Left of the top of the operating table stands the main monitoring rack. It presents waveforms of the electrocardiogram and three invasive blood pressures on an analogue screen. Up to 6 derived variables such as heart rate, systolic/mean/diastolic values and also temperatures can be presented by means of LED (light-emitting diode) displays placed lower in the rack. This same set of waveforms and variables is also presented on a slave monitor positioned high on the far wall of the operating room (OR). At the left of the main monitoring rack an 8-channel strip chart recorder has been positioned with the cardiac output computer on top. The value of the cardiac output is presented on a small LED display and a small recorder is incorporated to show the thermodilution curve. A ventilator has been placed to the right of the top of the table . The ventilator is equipped with rather a diversity of controls, dials and LED dis-

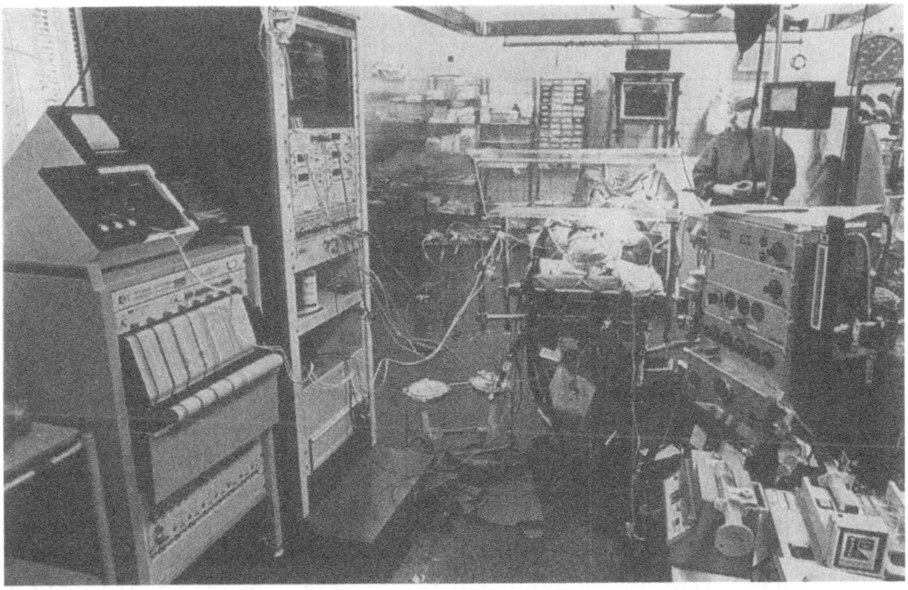

Fig. 1.4 An operating room for cardiac surgery (1983). The equipment to be used by the anesthesiologist is sophisticated. However, the level of uniformity and integration is low. The setup makes a cluttered impression.

plays, the height of which is sometimes so minimal that kneeling is required. The top of the ventilator is used as a writing tableau. More equipment is placed on this side such as a CO_2 analyzer, infusion pumps and the cart with drugs, bandages, etc. The positioning of the CPB apparatus is too far away to enable monitoring by the anesthesiologist. In short: in a situation which entails more risk for the patient than flying in an airplane the surveyability of the equipment is way below the standard of that in an airplane cockpit.

2 The Anesthesiologist's Work in the Operating Room

2.1 Introduction

In this chapter we will elaborate on a part of the knowledge which is required to determine whether and how the current concept of DADS should be improved to make DADS function as an optimal aid in monitoring by the anesthesiologist.

In Chapter 4 where the evaluation method is described, we will derive the subjects on which this knowledge, necessary for detecting these problems, is required. It will follow that the basic knowledge is of an organizing character:

- How well is the layout of the operating room adjusted to the task of the anesthesiologist?
- How often are certain data used for decision making by the anesthesiologists?
- How much time does the anesthesiologist spend on specific tasks?
- How efficiently can the monitoring and controlling function be performed?
- How often do certain mistakes (or near mistakes) occur and how critical is such a mistake? etc.

This chapter deals mainly with the first four points mentioned above. The organization of anesthesia management will be considered from various angles. This broad approach has the consequence that the character of the collected information is not of the type from which solutions can always be immediately obtained. It provides us with a *framework* in which the problems can be indicated. A next step is to determine whether realization of an improvement is possible and useful to DADS. Then further research must be done to effectuate realization. In conclusion this chapter will lead to a number of recommendations for improvements in the OR and in anesthesia management. Some of these recommendations will be elaborated upon in later chapters.

First, in Section 2.2, a global description of the task of the anesthesiologist will be given. In the subsequent sections the "framework-oriented knowledge" will be collected. In Section 2.3 the various layouts of operating rooms will be considered. This will be followed by a section in which the task of the anesthesiologist is considered from the point of view the way his work is organized; the fluctuations and differences in workload for specific subtasks and interactions between the various tasks of the team members will be discussed.

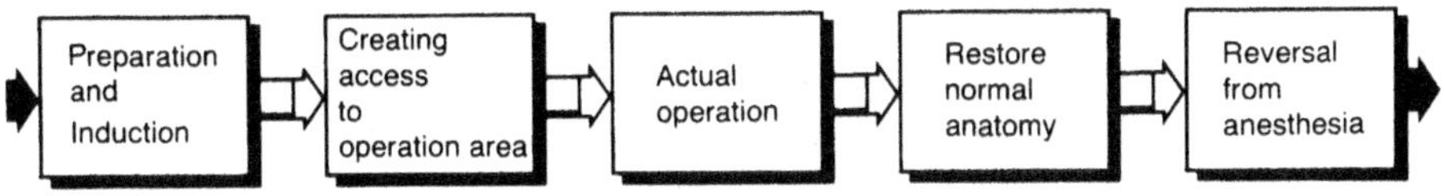

Fig. 2.1 The five main phases of a surgical procedure

2.2 General Task Description

During the course of cardiac surgery the patient is submitted to a number of drastic medical interventions related to the three main surgical phases of any operation (Fig. 2.1):

- creation of access to the area to be operated upon
- the actual operation
- restoration of the normal anatomy

The most common cardiac surgery procedures are:

- Coronary bypass procedures in which one or more obstructions in coronary arteries are bypassed by attaching grafts with one end to the root of the aorta and with the other end(s) distal to the obstruction
- Correction of congenital cardiac vitia
- Replacement of valves

In this text the expression "cardiac surgical procedures" refers to coronary bypass procedures. To enable the execution of an operation, the state of the patient has to meet a number of requirements. To bring, keep and reverse the patient into, in, and from this patho-physiological state is the task of the anesthesiologist.

Guidelines for patient care in anesthesiology as amended by the House of Delegates in the US are given in an ASA newsletter (1985). Dripps et al. (1982) described the task of the anesthesiologist during surgery as follows:

"The principal tasks of the anesthesiologist are to provide relief from pain for patients during operation and optimal operative conditions for surgeons, both in the safest possible manner. To do this the anesthesiologist must be a competent physician and a clinical pharmacologist, with a broad knowledge of surgery and the ability to utilize and interpret correctly a variety of devices [for monitoring and maintenance of vital functions]".

The induction and maintenance of anesthesia require the use of drugs which all result, in varying degrees, in the following:

- Narcosis (sleep)
- Analgesia (pain suppression)
- Amnesia (memory suppression)
- Suppression of autonomic responses
- Muscle relaxation

All drugs are potentially toxic. Therefore the "art" of anesthesiology is to balance on the edge of what is required and what can be considered as the minimum amount of drugs needed to realize, in the best interest of the patient, sufficient narcosis, analgesia and amnesia and loss of autonomic responses while providing sufficient muscle relaxation and loss of autonomic responses to allow the work of the surgeon to proceed in an optimal way. Thus it is not the surgery alone which causes many disturbances of the vital functions of the patient: the same applies to the anesthesia. Both specialties have in common that, though their goal is to improve the patient's condition, they are a threat in themselves.

One important example of a life-threatening intervention is the complete relaxation of the respiratory muscles, required to enable operation within the thoracic cavity. Respiration has then to be taken care of by using a ventilator, the control of which also belongs to the task of the anesthesiologist.

A definition of monitoring can be found in Webster's Dictionary (1979): "Monitoring is to observe and watch for a special purpose". The special purpose in this case involves the continuous assessment of a patient's condition, with emphasis on detection of changes (Dripps et al. 1982, p76).

The task of the anesthesiologist can be presented in a control loop (Fig. 2.2) which includes a permanent monitoring function. During monitoring, the anesthesiologist obtains information regarding the state of a patient via two routes: from 1) direct clinical observations (signs) and 2) equipment connected to the patient (signals). This information is compared with the desired state of the patient and it is decided whether (additional) medical interventions are necessary.

For various surgical procedures the same clinical observations are maintained, including:

skin color
skin temperature
pupil size *
perspiration *
lacrimation *
eye movements/small *
twitches in the face *
limb movements *
blood color

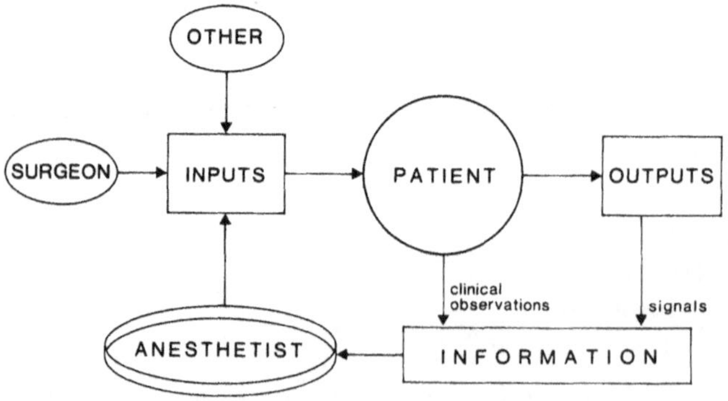

Fig. 2.2 The decision making of the anesthesiologist is based on directly and indirectly obtained data.

urinary output
fluid loss
respiratory movements

Where asterisks designate the signs indicating depth of anesthesia.

The number and type of observations which are to be maintained on signals from the applied equipment depend strongly on the type of procedure and the state of the patient. According to Saidman and Smith (1984, p80):

"The need for monitoring can be related to the predictability of the events associated with anesthesia and surgery. Patients with preexisting diseases such as hypertension or coronary artery disease, especially those undergoing complex sur-

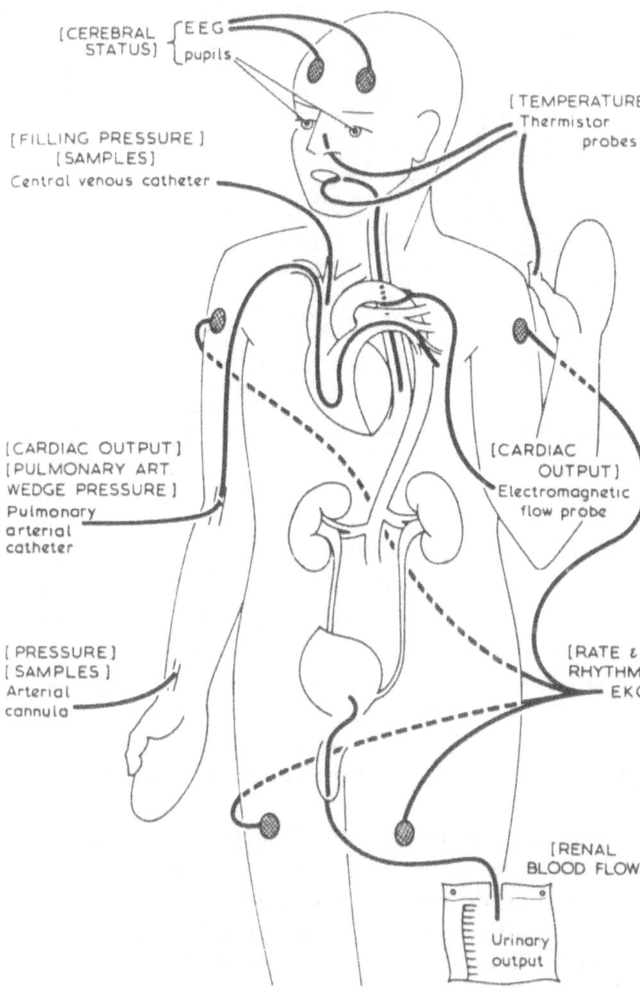

Fig. 2.3 The catheters and electrodes attached to the body. The EEG is not (yet?) a standard measurement during cardiac surgery. (From Gerson GR ed (1981) *Monitoring during anesthesia.* By permission of Little, Brown and Co.)

gery involving major blood loss and replacement, behave in a very unpredictable manner. More complex and invasive monitoring is then justified."

In the following we will give a short explanation of the main, indirectly obtained signals which are monitored during cardiac surgery (Fig. 2.3) with respect to their current use in the OR.

The Electrocardiogram (ECG): The electrical activity of the heart is reflected in the ECG, which is presented as an analogue waveform on a screen. The ECG is a quasi-periodical signal. During cardiac surgery it is generally measured by means of 4 electrodes attached at positions depending on the character of the operation and the wish to observe specific changes of interest. For example, it is deemed important that a shift in the ST segment be detected early because it may indicate ischemia of the myocardium. A review of the possible changes in the rhythm of the ECG is presented by Meijler et al. (1975). The heart rate (HR) is the number of periods per minute as derived from the ECG and is presented in numeric form.

The HR is watched closely to detect:

- bradycardia (which can be caused by too strong a reaction to the anesthetics for instance at induction)
- tachycardia (which can be caused by stress and pain reactions, for instance at sternotomy, mediastinal dissection, etc.)
- pacemaker functioning of the sinus node
- and, of course, to prevent cardiac arrest.

HR and ECG waveforms are observed to detect the incidence of ventricular extrasystoles, which may precede ventricular tachycardia, sometimes leading to ventricular fibrillation. Furthermore, the ECG is watched closely before and during cardioplegia, while going on bypass and while reactivating the heart at weaning from bypass.

Arterial Pressure (PART): One of the main regulatory mechanisms of the cardiovascular system is to maintain systemic arterial pressure within a tightly constrained range (Saidman and Smith 1984, p81). Therefore, it is sensible to use changes in the arterial pressure as a means of monitoring circulation.

PART is measured by means of an invasive catheter usually located in one of the radial arteries. The analogue waveform is presented and used initially to judge the reliability of the recorded signal.

When the signal is judged to be correct, parameters of the signal can be reliably derived.

The systolic arterial pressure (PSYS) is presented in digital form and monitored mainly to detect stress/pain and a possible increase in systemic vascular resistance. Multiplied by HR it is sometimes used as an indication of myocardial oxygen consumption, although it is also influenced by many more factors, such as contractility and ventricular wall tension. The diastolic arterial pressure (PDIA) is used to provide some kind of a check on the adequacy of myocardial perfusion.

The mean arterial pressure (MAP) is computed from the PART waveform. MAP reflects the driving pressure pushing blood into the system. Invasively measured, the MAP is less sensitive to artifacts of the measuring system than PSYS (Gravenstein and Paulus 1982, p44). The slope of the upstroke of the PART waveform is considered an indication of the contractility of the heart. In Ream (1982, pp156,157) exact and elaborate information may be found regarding the use of a combination of several hemodynamic variables for the control of physiological behavior under clinical conditions.

Central Venous Pressure (CVP) and Pulmonary Arterial Pressure (PAP): CVP is measured by means of a catheter in the jugular vein with its tip positioned in or near the right atrium. If the waveform is correct, the derived mean central venous pressure (MCVP) is used as a measure of right ventricular filling pressure.

If medically indicated, that is when right heart signals do not give enough information about left heart functioning, a so-called pulmonary arterial catheter is applied. This is introduced through the jugular or another vein; by means of a small balloon at the tip of the catheter it can be floated into the pulmonary artery. Through the sensor at the tip of this catheter the PAP can be measured continuously. The balloon at the tip of the catheter can be insufflated a number of times during a cardiac procedure. In this way, a branch of the pulmonal artery can be occluded and pulmonary arterial wedge pressure (PAWP) is measured. PAWP is used as an estimation for the left ventricular end diastolic pressure (LVEDP). This is possible because there are no valves between the pulmonary artery and the left atrium and because of the anatomy of the pulmonary vascular bed.

Cardiac Output (CO): Through an additional entrance port in the pulmonary arterial catheter a cold solution can be injected to determine the CO by means of the thermodilution method (van der Werf 1965); this measurement is usually performed 4 times during a procedure but, because the measurement has a low reproducibility due to influences of, among other things, respiration (Stetz et al. 1982), the average of three actual measurements is needed each time.

CO is used to check the overall functioning of the heart and also to resolve doubts as to whether a low PART is caused by a low CO or by vasodilation etc.

Based on CO and other available data a whole range of derived variables can be computed such as the systemic vascular resistance (SVR=(MAP-MCVP)/CO).

A useful decision table regarding inferences which can be made from CVP and CO with respect to effective blood volume is given by Gravenstein and Paulus (1982, p130). Fogdall (1982, pp465,467) presents a decision table regarding the correction of a low CO and of a high CO in combination with the state of the MAP.

Core and Skin Temperature (Tcore and Tskin): Tcore is generally measured in the nasopharynx and Tskin at the toe. In the absence of the means to determine CO, their difference is sometimes used to assess the adequacy of peripheral perfusion.

Furthermore, their difference is important for checking the cooling and rewarming processes inherent to the bypass period. During bypass Tskin will be higher than Tcore because cooling takes place from the center of the patient.

Ventilation signals (VENT): The type of ventilator applied determines which are the parameters to be either adjusted (inputs) or measured at the ventilator (outputs). Most important are the volume of gas expired per minute (MIVOL), the respiratory rate (RRATE), the maximal inspiratory pressure (PRMX), and of course the settings of inspired O_2 and N_2O.

Capnogram (CO_2): CO_2 is usually sampled through a catheter that is inserted into the anesthesia circuit close to the patient's mouth (Gravenstein and Paulus 1982, p159). Peters (1979) formulates the advantages of CO_2 measurement as follows: "A monitor that can track in real time the concentration of CO_2 in the in- and expired air [permits], as no other signal can, the [supervision] of both the ventilatory and the metabolic systems. In addition, in patients with normal pulmonary function, the end-expired PCO_2 is a reflection of the arterial PCO_2 and thus of adequacy of cell respiration". The capnogram is monitored to detect a disconnected ventilator, problems with oxygenation when inspired O_2 is not measured, pulmonary embolization, hyperventilation or hypoventilation (e.g. from obstruction in airway), but also abnormal blood flow in the lung.

Many possible changes in the capnogram and their causes are described in an atlas composed by Smalhout and Kalenda (1975). Ream (1982, pp468,469) gives decision tables for respiratory management of arterial PO_2 and PCO_2 and of bicarbonate.

Discussion: The adequacy of decision making depends, primarily, on the concepts and quality of the (signal) monitoring.

When considering the monitoring task (with respect to the signals) from a medical viewpoint, it should be noted that the following problems may occur:

- The quality of the signal may not be sufficient. For blood pressures this may be due to problems with the introduction of a catheter, to clotting during the procedure, or to a slight shift in the position of the catheter, causing it to lie against the wall of the vessel. Also, the transfer characteristics of a catheter may be adversely affected by tiny air bubbles in the line, causing damping of the waveform. In all these cases the signal can not be trusted and what is worse it may even remain unnoticed that the signal quality is insufficient (Plasman 1981, de Beer 1984, v Rijswijk 1986).
- An insufficient quality of ECG and temperature signals is quite often caused by ill-connected electrodes/sensors. Besides, the quality of the ECG may be strongly impaired by the electrocautery signal. Periodic variations, such as from respiration, may influence the reproducibility of values such as cardiac output and diastolic pulmonary pressure (Yelderman et al. 1980).
- The efficacy of monitoring also depends on the parameters included in the monitoring. The risk to the patient caused by an additional monitoring device (catheter) should always be weighed against the additional value to the quality of monitoring. For example the decision to use the pulmonary arterial catheter should always be taken with great care (Kaplan 1983).
- Another indistinctness concerns the subject of derived variables; there is a never-ending discussion about the additional value/redundancy of these, for example: when systolic and diastolic pressures are determined, what is the contribution of the mean arterial pressure?

- An additional problem area is the continuous stream of "new" parameters which can be measured in the operating room. These include, at the moment, the electroencephalogram and its derived parameters, transcutaneous or invasive measurement of oxygen saturation, the electromyogram and new plethysmographic techniques.

In most cases the problems mentioned above are recognized and are made the subject of investigation by anesthesiologists. In this book we shall not tackle these problems but consider the organization of information presentation and transfer in the OR as far as it concerns the work of the anesthesiologist.

2.3 The Operating Room: Layout, Equipment, and Information Presentation

In this section layout, equipment and information presentation in some operating rooms for cardiac surgery will be discussed.

Possible indications for necessary improvements in DADS should not only be found in the current functioning and facilities of DADS itself but the operating room as a whole should be investigated to come to a revision of DADS with respect to information presentation, transfer and control. Besides, it is important to ensure that DADS is not being adjusted to the situation in only one particular operating room but is designed to be generally applicable.

To get an idea of the differences and resemblances in operating rooms, we studied the monitoring situation in 7 operating rooms which we were able to visit (Fig. 2.4). In most operating rooms the equipment is similarly arranged:

1 In the center, the operating table
2 At the side of the operating table (sometimes straight sometimes awry), leaving room for the surgeons, the cardiopulmonary bypass apparatus
3 Directly to the left or the right from the head of the operating table, the ventilator and the anesthesia delivery machine
4 Directly near the head of the patient, the transducers for invasive blood pressure measurement. The leads originating from these transducers are attached to a rack for monitoring of hemodynamic variables, temperatures and ECG, which is positioned near the anesthesiologist. Signals from this rack are sometimes transmitted to a recorder
5 Drip infusions slightly aside and above the head of the table; infusion pumps in most cases at a distance less than one meter
6 The cautery apparatus and the defibrillator to be used by the surgeons have various locations
7 Additional (special) equipment
8 The cart, positioned within easy reach of the anesthesiologist

The observed deviations from the general layout outlined above were as follows:

ad 3.

- The ventilator is accommodated to take care of the delivery of gases and volatiles (OK5,6,7).

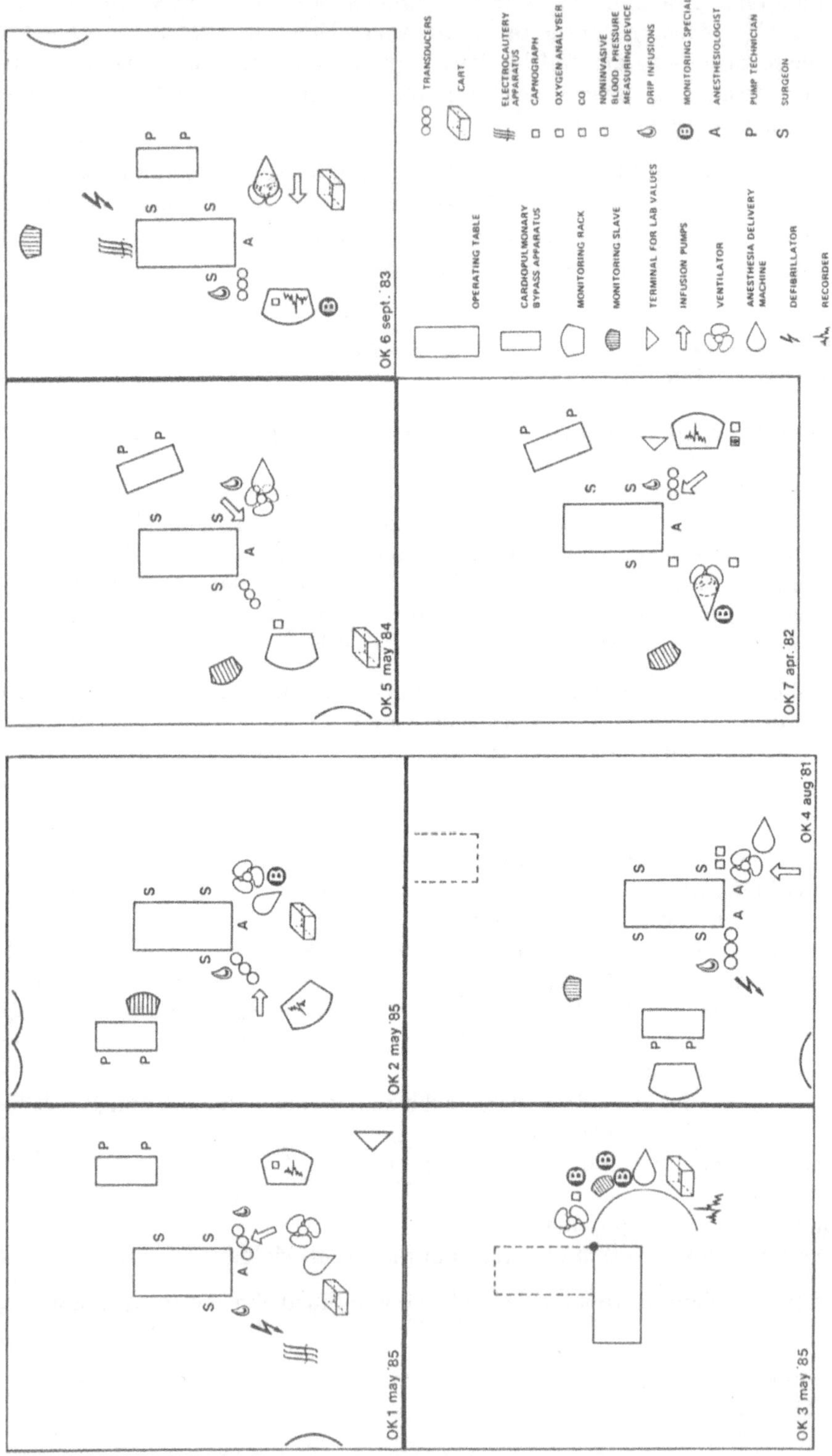

Fig. 2.4 Drafts which have been made of 7 operating rooms to illustrate the nonuniformity and nonintegration in the setup of the equipment. An explanatory list for the symbols used in the drafts has been included.

- The ventilator and the anesthesia delivery apparatus are spatially separated (OK3).

ad 4.

- The central monitoring rack does not present both analogue signals (waveforms) and digital values, but only the waveforms (OK1).
- The central monitoring rack includes trend plotting and is provided with an alarm algorithm which is (meant) to be more sophisticated than the common static alarm system (OK5).
- There is no multi-channel recorder (OK4). The recorder is not incorporated in the monitoring rack (OK3,5), or is positioned outside the OR (OK5).
- There is no slave to the central monitor (OK1,3), thus the positioning of the central monitor is (must be) such that it can be seen by the whole team.
- The slave is fixed near the pump technicians (OK2). The monitoring rack is placed a little behind the anesthesiologists (OK1,2,3).
- The CO computer is incorporated in the central monitoring rack (OK1,6).

ad 7.

- Blood gas values and electrolytes are automatically presented on a terminal or printer in the OR (OK1,7).
- Inspired and expired gas concentrations are measured continuously by means of a mass spectrometer positioned outside the operating room; results are presented in the operating room on a special monitor (OK2,3).
- Special displays are available for presentation of combinations of variables by means of alternative formats (OK6,7). Additional facilities are available for computation of specific derived variables (OK6,7), or for additional higher-level alarming (OK6).
- A plotter is available for the generation of an automated anesthesia record (OK3,6).

When we consider the operating rooms with their equipment setups as described above and with their respective layouts, we observe the following aspects as being positive:

All facilities as mentioned under point 7 are useful. In fact it should become standard practice that blood gas values and electrolytes are transmitted and presented in the operating room on a terminal or printer without actions being required from the staff in the operating room.

An advantage of determining in- and expired gas concentrations by means of a mass spectrometer is that especially the inspired concentration is known with greater precision and that practically continuous (trend) monitoring is possible (Sodal and Swanson 1980). This enhances the speedy recognition of changes. A cheaper and also adequate solution for analyzing the gas components could be the use of separate infrared devices.

Automatic generation of an anesthesia record considerably reduces the workload of the anesthesiologist and improves the accuracy of the record (Section 2.4 and Chapter 7).

Centralized and comprehensive presentation of data on a single display instead of on distributed displays may also enhance decision making (Chapters 3 and 5).

Apart from these items under point 7, the surveyable semi-circular arrangement of equipment as in OK3 constitutes a positive attempt at integration. However, it has the disadvantage that most of the equipment is positioned behind the anesthesiologist. This disadvantage is resolved in OK1 by entrusting an additional nurse with the scanning of the monitoring rack.

A potentially dangerous situation - the possibility of the anesthesiologist tripping over badly arranged transducer leads cluttering his workspace - was provisionally solved in OK2 by bundling the leads in a flexible plastic tube.

In OK7 the confusion which often occurs with respect to which transducer(port) belongs to which catheter is obviated by applying a color code to transducer ports and leads.

OK3 is part of a very advanced project of central hospital automation. A so-called anesthesia information and management system (AIMS) is being developed (Frazier 1985 priv. comm.). This system bridges the gap between the administrative network within the hospital and the medical departments. Medical data on every procedure which the patient undergoes, is entered into a computer. Any previously stored information of interest for an ongoing procedure can be retrieved.

A more sophisticated alarm algorithm as applied in OK5 and OK6 may be an (as yet to be tested) improvement over the common means of alarm generation in the operating room which are mostly audible alarms triggered when the static limits are exceeded.

Conclusion: Though practically the same variables are monitored and controlled in the various ORs, this uniformity does not hold for the equipment and its positioning in relation to these tasks.

As yet, positive new acquisitions such as trend presentation, mass spectrometers and automated transfer of lab data are applied only on an individualistic basis. Less surprisingly, this is also true for more experimental facilities such as sophisticated alarms and automated record keeping. Above, we used the differences between the ORs to determine both weak points and recommendable positive points in the layout. Points suitable for implementation in systems like DADS will be elaborated upon later.

2.4 Flowcharting Anesthesia

Apart from the considerations above, an analysis of the organization of the task of the anesthesiologist in the operating room may provide us with further starting points for improvement (Gravenstein et al. 1970). Conspicuous aspects of the functioning are the necessary interaction with so many other team members and the fluctuation in workload. With respect to the latter, flurries of energetic activity alternate with periods of boredom; with respect to the former, a team of about 11 members has to cooperate during a cardiac surgical procedure (Fig. 2.5).

Such a team usually consists of two surgeons. A third surgeon is in attendance during bypass operations with the task of preparing vessels from the leg, which have to be used as grafts. A surgical nurse has the task of assisting with the opera-

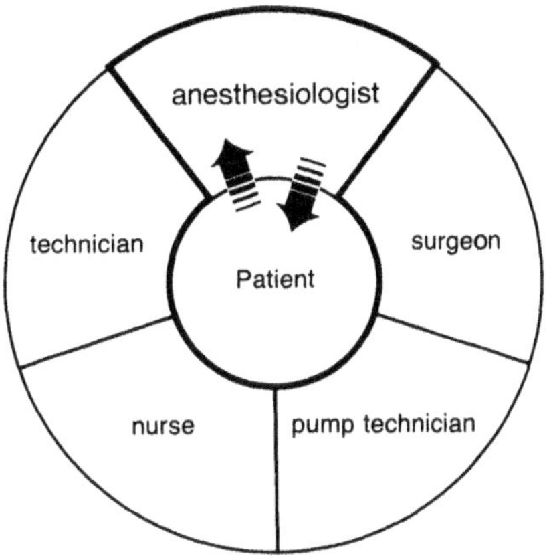

Fig. 2.5 The considerable staff required at a cardiac surgical procedure is a complicating factor for the task performance of the anesthesiologist.

Table 2.1 The 9 activity codes for anesthesia management according to Kennedy et al. (1976). Permission granted by the Int. Anesth. Research Soc.

Symbol	Description	Attention*
ACI	Adjust or calibrate instrument (respirator, heating blanket, IV)	T&A
AW	Arrange equipment (instruments, table)	A
DT	Data transfer : anesthetist communicates or gestures to another person	A
LDC	Log data on anesthetic record or read chart	A
MAD	Mix or administer drugs	T
OIS	Observe oscilloscope or other monitor	T
OP	Observe patient (skin color, surgical field, etc.)	T
PP	Prepare patient (place ECG leads, BP, transducers, etc.)	T
SA	Scan area (attention not directed to any instruments or display but scanning entire field)	T

* "T" indicates that the anesthetist's attention is directed *toward* the patient-surgical field. "A" indicates that the anesthetist's attention is directed *away* from the patient-surgical field.

tion and passing the instruments. A number of nurses are in attendance to supply the sterile implements, to weigh the soaked surgical sponges and to fill in the surgical record. The CPB apparatus is, in most cases, manned by two pump technicians. Anesthesia is mostly administered by one anesthesiologist assisted by an anesthetics nurse. Sometimes a second anesthesiologist is in attendance. Outside the operating room a technician is on standby in case of technical problems. The extensiveness of such a team asks for advanced interaction facilities, but until now not much attention has been given to this subject.

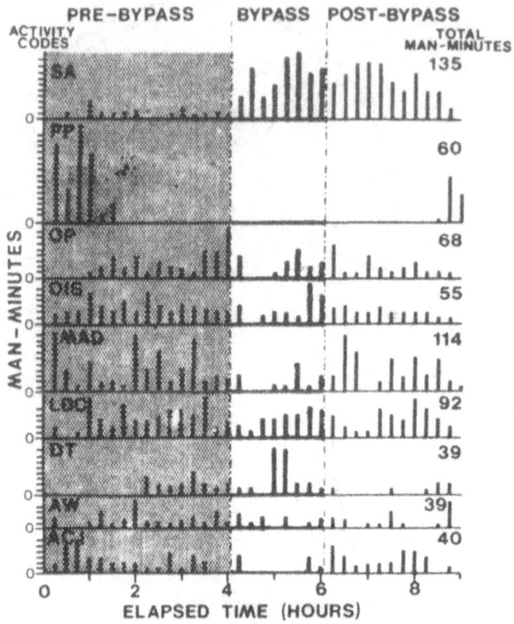

Fig. 2.6 An illustration of the chronological workload of the anesthesiologist. Man-minutes expended during 15-minute periods on 9 activities during one procedure are given. Note at induction the peaks in Prepare Patient, Mix and Administer Drugs and Adjust and Calibrate Instruments. Note the increase in activity at going from bypass and toward the end of the procedure. From Kennedy et al. (1976). Permission granted by the Int. Anesth. Research Soc.

In order to study the division of the time spent by the anesthesiologist, we refer to two papers in which anesthesia management was recorded by means of video cameras: the actions were classified and the time spent on each subtask was determined by counting the frames dedicated to the various tasks (Kennedy et al. 1976, Boquet et al. 1980).

Kennedy et al. (1976) applied this method during three coronary bypass procedures with a duration of 6, 8 and 9 hours. (Currently the average duration of bypass procedures is shorter. However, this does not seem to influence markedly the relative time division.) The management was divided into 9 subtasks (Table 2.1) and frame length was fixed at 2 seconds. The authors give, per procedure, the time spent in man-minutes on every subtask. For one operation they also present, per subtask, the chronological fluctuations in workload (Fig. 2.6).

Boquet et al. (1980) analyzed 15 general (noncardiac) surgical procedures by means of separate filming of manual and visual activities (frame length 0.5 sec). The aim of this study was to design a new anesthesia delivery machine according to human engineering concepts. Therefore they applied a subdivision corresponding at most points with the various pieces of equipment. This subdivision is not equal to the task division as used by Kennedy et al. (1976).

To be able to make comparisons between the workload as determined in the two studies, the subdivision as applied by Boquet has been converted to the subdi-

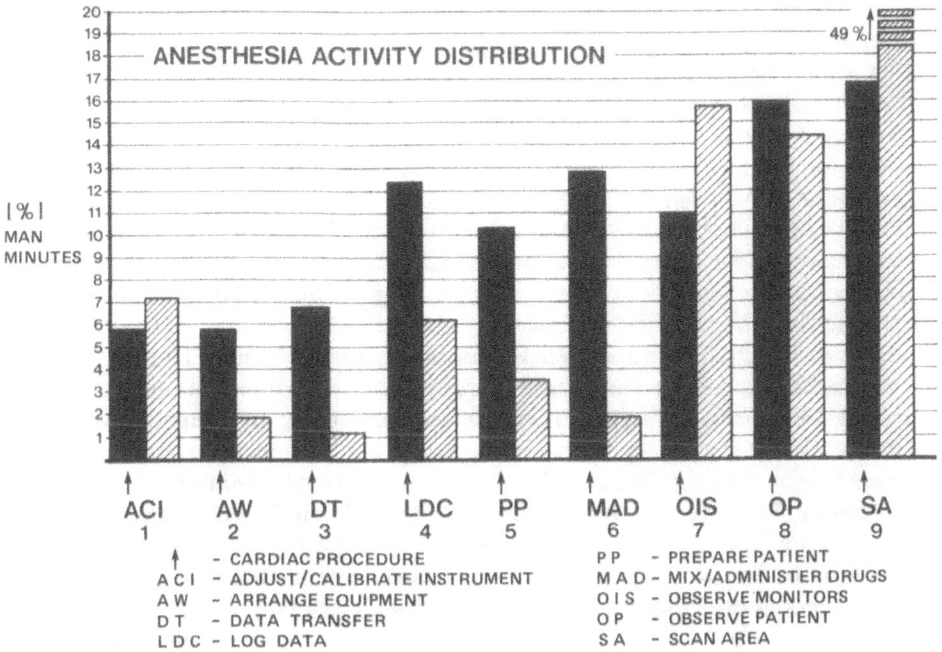

Fig. 2.7 In this figure the only available quantitative material on anesthesia workload is presented. The time spent in percentage man-minutes on nine subtasks is plotted for cardiac surgical procedures (left columns) (after Kennedy et al. 1976) and for general procedures (right columns) (after Boquet et al. 1980).

vision by Kennedy and manual and visual activities are taken together. The resulting workload histogram is given in Fig. 2.7.

It is obvious that differences between the bypass (left) and general (right) procedures exist. During cardiac surgery more time has to be spent on certain subtasks (nos. 2,3,4,5,6) than during general procedures. On the other hand much less time is spent on, or even available for, the Scan Area task (no. 9) (17% vs. 48%). This confirms the general impression that cardiac anesthesia procedures are more work-intensive.

This is due to the following: In contrast to the mostly noninvasive techniques as used for general procedures, in cardiac surgery catheters and sensors are often employed. The introduction of the pulmonary arterial catheter is especially time-consuming (Prepare Patient).

Blood gas values and electrolytes are measured rather frequently during cardiac surgery and have to be recorded together with the repeated observations from a considerable number of monitors and of clinical signs (Log Data on Chart).

Apart from the medications applied for induction, cardiac anesthesia requires more: these include anesthetics to be administered just in advance of stress-arousing interventions such as sternotomy, intubation and the introduction of cannulas. Furthermore, continuous control of blood pressures, with vasoactive drugs and/or fluids, and of the cardiac output, by means of inotropic drugs, is often required (Mix and Administer Drugs).

The positioning of infusion pumps may require additional time apart from the sorting and clearing activities at the cart (Arrange Equipment).

A clear example of the necessary interaction between the surgeon and the anesthesiologist is the often trivial discussion regarding the positioning of the table: tilting may be required in order to facilitate the work of the surgeon.

Further interaction takes place between the anesthesiologist and the pump technician regarding the drugs to be administered during perfusion (Data Transfer).

During cardiac surgery relatively less time is spent on the observation of monitors. Apart from the heavier workload in other subtasks, this may be due to the period during which the aorta is clamped (duration about 40 min.). During this period the metabolic state of the patient is quite stable (hypothermia) and more area scanning takes place or delayed tasks such as data logging are caught up with. It is estimated that there are 5 periods during which the monitors are very intensively observed (priv. comm. v Wezel 1986) (Table 2.2) (Observe Monitors).

Following these general remarks we will elaborate on the suitability of the different subtasks for automation. The tasks 1,2,5,6 from Fig. 2.7 all require manual activities from the anesthesiologist. To automate parts of these we enter the field of automated control which is beyond the scope of this book.

The tasks which remain to be investigated with respect to their suitability for automation are:

ACI Adjust Instruments and Controls: Not only the information presentation in ORs is too decentralized: the handling of the equipment has also not been organized efficiently (Chapter 1). In Chapter 6 it will be shown that, by integrating the arrangement of equipment, an improvement can be realized.

DT Data Transfer: An important global task which is interwoven with the whole surgical procedure is the maintenance of the depth of anesthesia and the regulation of the circulation. During cardiac bypass surgery an additional special procedure is required:

There is a period during which surgical manipulations are performed on the heart itself and the pumping activity of the heart is suppressed. To this end the CPB apparatus (or heart-lung machine) is applied (Fig. 2.8). By means of two cannulas, deoxygenated blood is drained from the Venae cavae superior and inferior. Next, the blood is oxygenated in the machine and subsequently returned to the body via a third cannula which is placed in the aorta or a femoral artery. In this

Table 2.2 Phases and duration of intensive signal monitoring

catheterization	5 min
induction	10 min
incision&sternotomy	20 min
cannulation	5 min
weaning from bypass	30 min

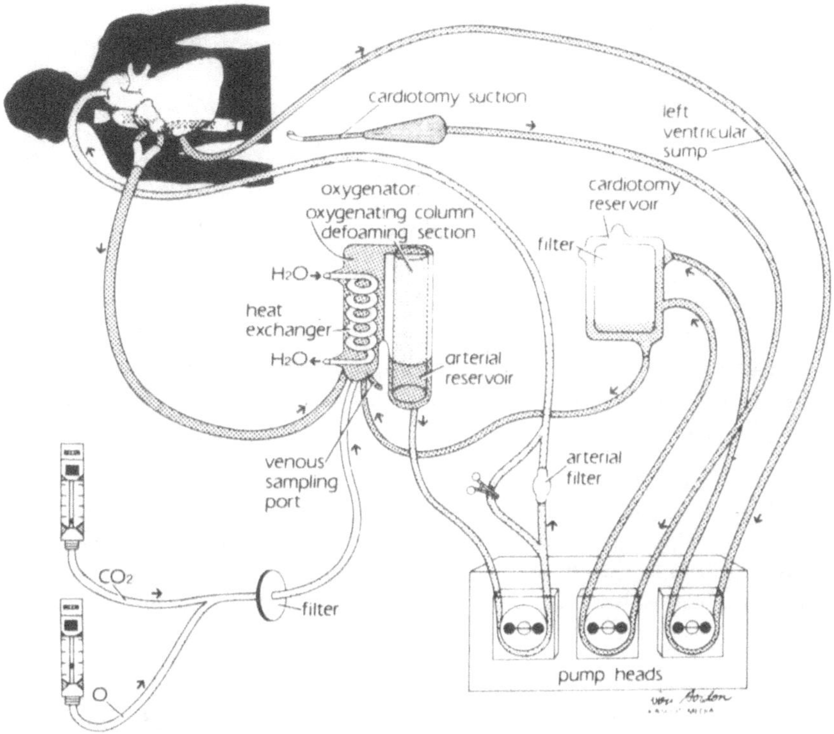

Fig. 2.8 Cardiopulmonary Bypass apparatus (CPB). The parameters controlled and presented on this apparatus are of importance for monitoring by the anesthesiologist. (From Dripps et al. 1972, Permission granted by WB Saunders, Philadelphia). Note the following: gravity drainage from venae cavae to oxygenator; heat exchanger with entrance and exit ports for water; separate sources for oxygen and carbon dioxide; left ventricular sump for decompression of left ventricle via right superior pulmonary vein with return of blood to oxygenator via cardiotomy reservoir; and arterial filter bypass in the event of filter obstruction.

way the oxygen supply to the body is maintained even after the heart is stopped. The heart is stopped by cooling the circulating blood in the CPB apparatus and by injecting a cardioplegic liquid in the coronary arteries.

During the period from start to stop bypass, not only circulation and oxygenation but also the administration of drugs and the sampling of blood for determination of blood gas values and electrolytes are regulated from the CPB apparatus. However, the responsibility of the anesthesiologist with respect to these actions is maintained. This results in a rather long period (1-1.5 hours) during which the anesthesiologist and the pump technician have shared responsibilities. As a result, interaction (data transfer) between anesthesiologist and pump technician is necessary and frequent. Apart from the hemodynamic signals as measured at the patient and displayed at slave and master monitors, during bypass the pump technician is supplied with additional information from the CPB apparatus. These variables are mentioned below and their value for the anesthesiologist is indicated with + and – signs.

Flow overall:
+ Comparable to CO, the amount of blood circulating round the body per minute.

Master-slave settings of rotor pumps:
– Master setting is sometimes adjusted at the request of the surgeon when he needs lower flow to operate or to identify anatomic details.

Height of the cardiotomy apparatus:
+ – The level of the cardiotomy apparatus is used to adjust the filling pressures of the patient.

Line pressure:
+ – A measure for the pressure with which the blood has to bridge the distance between the CPB apparatus and the body. Sometimes important to detect kinking of a cannula.

Shim pressure and O_2 Flow in:
– Increasing shim pressure means increased contact of the O_2 flow with the blood. Shim pressure and O_2 flow together determine the oxygen supply to the blood. The anesthesiologist is more interested in the resulting oxygenation as determined from blood gas values.

CO_2ex:
+ During bypass the pulsatile behavior of the capnogram such as normally measured near the mouth of the patient disappears. At the venous side of the oxygenator a non-pulsatile CO_2 level can now be used as a measure for ventilation and metabolism.

Bubbles:
– Exclusive responsibility of the pump technicians.

Filter pressures:
– Idem, these are important for detecting clotting and/or a pinched cannula.

Temperature of cooling water:
+ Important for speed of cooling and rewarming.

The setting of vaporizers for the administration of volatiles and the setting of infusion pumps for the administration of vasoactive drugs:
+ Medications influencing depth of anesthesia and circulation are the responsibility of the anesthesiologist.

Remaining administered medications such as heparin, antibiotics, intravenous anesthetics:
+ Idem

Start and stop of cardioplegia:
+ Of interest with respect to heart activity.

During bypass the so-called activated clotting time (ACT) of the blood must be extended to 800 seconds or more, in order to prevent clotting of the blood in cannulas and filters. This value is determined in a small appliance positioned near the

anesthesiologist; depending on its value heparin has to be supplied by the pump technician:
+ Of interest for the pump technician with regard to heparinization.

In short, the greater part of this information is more or less of importance for monitoring by both the pump technician and the anesthesiologist. However, the anesthesiologist in particular does not have these parameters continuously at his disposal, a shortcoming which is met by verbal transfer of messages between pump technician and anesthesiologist, which can easily lead to mistakes or omissions. With respect to the data transfer task a considerable improvement may be effected by means of automation; automated readout of the variables from the heart-lung machine springs to mind. In this way an organized display of such variables in the operating room becomes possible. A display facility near the anesthesiologist can be extended to provide the means for an exchange of quantitative (coded) messages between the anesthesiologist and the pump technician.

LDC Log Data on Chart: The logging of patient data in a so-called anesthesia record consumes about 12% of the time of the anesthesiologist. This means that, for an operation of 5 hours, 35 minutes are spent on writing. Writing itself is clearly a task where attention is diverted away from the patient; on the other hand it can be stated that writing down a value requires, initially an observation which subsequently enhances attention to the patient (Noel 1986).

In most cases, the quality of the written record is rather poor and could benefit from automation; there may be other ways to keep attention focused on the patient. The usefulness of an automated anesthesia record was confirmed in many different ways and DADS (Chapter 3) is suitable for the generation of such a record because of its data storage and retrieval capacity. Therefore it was decided to extend the DADS with such a facility (Chapter 7).

OIS Observe Instruments and Monitors: The presentation of data in ORs is not sufficiently organized (see Section 2.4). Besides, there is a lack of enhanced monitoring facilities such as trend presentation, sophisticated alarms and computation of derived variables. For many of these problems, solutions are provided by DADS (Chapter 3).

SA Scan Area: Even though "only" 17% of the time is left for the scanning of the area, it is acknowledged that the level of boredom can be considerable. When employing automation to improve the efficiency of the tasks of the anesthesiologist it is recommendable to reduce, as much as possible, the causes of boredom which may lead to a decrease in vigilance (Branton 1980). An almost indispensable means of estimating the sensitivity of a patient for the surgical manipulations and the administered drugs is the presentation of trends. Automation enables the anesthesiologist to create trend plots at choice. A quiet period is most suitable for doing this and in the meantime it enhances vigilance: (missed) signal changes can still be recognized (Chapter 3).

Above we have considered the various subtasks of the anesthesiologist with respect to their suitability and usefulness for automation as if they were independent. However, the state of the patient depends on medical interventions which may be performed by surgeons, anesthesiologists and pump technicians and this interdependence should be taken into consideration. To obtain an idea of the character and number of interventions and their dependence on time and person, an activity flowchart of anesthesia management was composed (Appendix 1.). In this scheme the anesthesia management takes the central position. Actions of the anesthesiologists, such as monitoring and administering drugs, are plotted against a global time scale. Many actions of the anesthesiologist are induced by preceding or subsequent actions of the surgeons; these are therefore placed in the first column of the scheme. The activities of the pump technicians and anesthetics nurse have been also included.

When, in the category "monitoring", signals are mentioned for the first time, this means that their monitoring has begun at that point. Subsequent reference means that the specific signal has been observed with special attentiveness. The main reason for which signals are observed is also given.

From this activity chart we can derive the list of standard events as occurring during a procedure (Appendix 2.). Furthermore we can see that there are actions of the anesthesiologist which occur only once (when everything proceeds smoothly), such as intubation and sternotomy, and there are actions which are performed repeatedly, such as the determination of ACT (approx. 8 times), CO determination (4·3 times), blood sampling (approx. 7 times), ventilator adjustment (at least 5 times), reading of urinary output (3 times). There are also actions which consist of a sequence of smaller handlings such as preparing patient for bed, clearing cart etc.

The following remarks as to the efficiency of actions in the activity chart can be made:

A seemingly trivial problem is the determination of the urine production. Normally this must be done in three phases: before, towards the end, and well after bypass. However, it appears that the chance of an omission is considerable and it would be an improvement to automate the necessary actions.

A more complex problem is presented by the ergonomic properties of the ventilators. For instance in OK 6 the adjustment of the volatile agents knob on the vaporizer easily gives rise to mistakes: on and off settings can be mixed up and also the adjustment of O_2/N_2O mixtures may cause errors. This supports the opinion that the only exact monitoring of these settings is provided by the application of a mass spectrometer or several other gas analyzers.

The monitoring of drip infusions is susceptible to improvement.

The computation of settings from infusion pumps from mg/kg/h to ml/h and the computation of derived variables from, for instance the CO, is a recurrent necessity even when time is not available to perform these calculations. Computers are the solution to a problem like this.

2.5 Conclusions

By studying the organization of information presentation and transfer with respect to anesthesia management, a number of shortcomings have been revealed. Though some of them may appear to be rather trivial, it is just the concurrency of these awkward items which may well and indeed do give rise to adverse incidents (Chapter 8). Therefore, it is useful to apply the possibilities of automation in such a way that more practical order and structure in anesthesia management will be the result. The points on which improvements are recommended are summarized below and the way in which they were detected is indicated (OK = layouts, HIS = histogram subtasks, FLOW = activity chart):

In- and expired gases should be determined with a mass spectrometer (or more simply with analyzers providing about the same information) and presented in a centralized fashion. OK

Values of blood gases and electrolytes should automatically be transferred to the operating room and presented centrally. OK

Signal transfer from patient to front end equipment should be improved. One or zero cable transmission should be striven for (van der Vorst 1985). OK

Attuning, more uniformity, and possibly integration of the anesthesia equipment should be obtained. (Chapter 6) OK

Centralized acquisition and easily surveyable display of all the currently presented patient signals should be realized. (Chapter 3) OK

It should be possible to couple DADS to the hospital information system, so that easy transfer of patient data from one system to another is possible. OK

Automated presentation of ventilator, perfusor and other settings on the data display equipment should be included in centralized information presentation. (partly Chapter 3) FLOW

Centralized alarms and shopping lists for all parameters, including empty infusion bottles (Downing 1983) and pumps, should be provided for. (partly Chapter 3) FLOW

Automated urine output determination would be useful (Shubin 1971). FLOW

Apart from centralized information presentation centralized equipment control is also necessary. (Chapter 6) OK

An automated anesthesia record would be a useful facility. (Chapter 7) HIS

Automated readout of parameters at the heart-lung machine, enabling their surveyable presentation, visible for both the pump technician and the anesthesiologist, would complete the variables which are to be monitored by the anesthesiologist. Possibly, a means for (coded) message interaction between these team members could be added. HIS

In close discussions with anesthesiologists we developed the DADS to be described in the next chapter. The goal was to realize a solution to one of the problems mentioned above, namely centralized acquisition and surveyable display of all the currently presented patient signals and also to solve part of one other problem, namely the alarming. In developing DADS it was clear that there are many more problems in ORs which may be solved by automation. In this chapter quite a few have been identified. Others will follow in the subsequent chapters.

3 The Data Acquisition and Display System (DADS)

3.1 Introduction

In the previous chapter a framework has been sketched of factors which may lead to adverse incidents in anesthesia. Some of these factors referred to information processing and transfer. The DADS described in this chapter was developed to improve matters in this respect (Fig. 3.1).

DADS is an intermediate station in a philosophy with regard to automation in anesthesia, as developed by Beneken and Blom (1983).

This philosophy can be illustrated by means of the so-called Magical Monitoring Matrix (Fig. 3.2). This matrix indicates the degree of signal processing and the kind of data presentation deemed necessary in relation to the number of signals included in monitoring.

In the first row the number of signals which may be monitored is indicated. During cardiac anesthesia this number may indeed be considerable (Section 2.2). In the first column the different signal processing methods are given in order of increasing complexity. Each is meant to enable alarming upon undesirable signal changes; the "ultimate" algorithm should enable state prediction, which in turn may lead to automatic control of (some) signals (servoanesthesia). In principle there are an infinite number of possibilities for signal processing, but this does not necessarily mean that an adequate signal processing algorithm can be designed.

The main problem is to prevent an algorithm from generating too many false alarms. One of the conditions for this is that the system must be able to account for the medical interventions (inputs). The algorithm can then relate the inputs to the signal behavior (outputs) and thus, alarms for expected changes or artifacts may be filtered out or prevented.

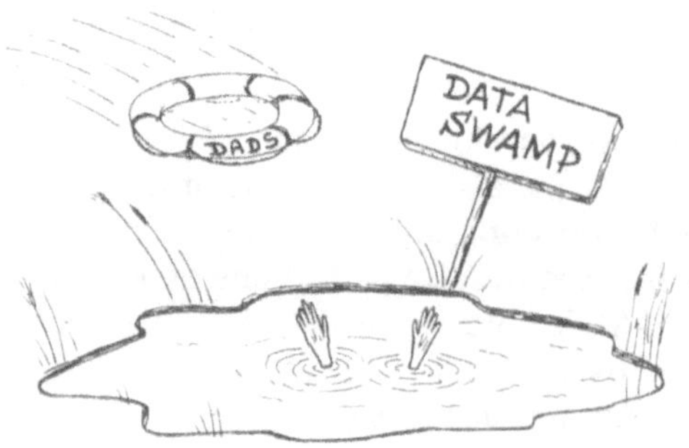

Fig. 3.1 DADS is meant to prevent the anesthesiologist from drawning in a swamp of data.

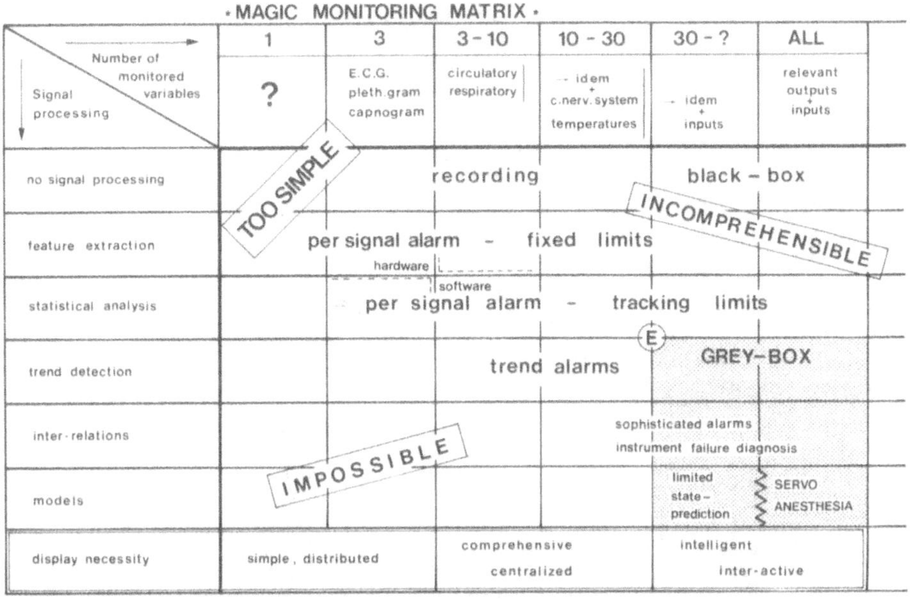

Fig. 3.2 The magical monitoring matrix (Beneken and Blom 1983) gives a comprehensive view of their philosophy regarding automation in anesthesia. Monitoring with only a few signals which are not processed will be too simple for most anesthetic procedures. The monitoring of about 30 signals without further processing is incomprehensible. To try to extract features from only a few signals by means of advanced signal processing is impossible. Adequate monitoring can only be achieved when the sophistication of signal processing and display increases with the number of variables included.

With its current alarm algorithm and data presentation DADS can be localized at the point in the Matrix marked with an E.

In Beneken's philosophy the ultimate objective is servoanesthesia. Therefore DADS as such is not only the goal of the project but also a means of obtaining that goal. Because of its capacity for continuous data storage, DADS can be used to collect and chart knowledge regarding decision making in anesthesia. In this way we may come a step nearer to the realization of a patient model which is necessary for the application of servoanesthesia.

For this reason one of the subobjectives during the evaluation of DADS has been the charting of clinically significant signal behavior during anesthesia. Along these lines some of the most important signal characteristics to which attention is paid during cardiac anesthesia were mentioned in Chapter 2.

In Chapter 5 the evaluation tests of DADS will also serve to obtain more knowledge about clinically significant signal changes.

The idea of computer-assisted monitoring is not new. In the 1960s, developments for application in *intensive care units* were initiated. Crul and Payne (1970) formulated the advantages of computer assisted monitoring as follows:

"Patient monitoring systems serve three main functions.

First they protect the patient by ensuring that variations in a physiological variable beyond an acceptable range are immediately apparent to the attendant clinician; secondly, they indicate the pattern of response to treatment so that it can be modified as required; and thirdly, they provide data from which advances in therapeutics may be developed".

Beaumont 19.. gives another formulation:

"At one level the attempt is to automate what a person can do as well, or better, on the basis that the computer is tireless and never inattentive or bored. It is generally in this area that one hopes to find cost-effectiveness in the sense that the same quality of care can be provided more economically by the elimination or minimization of staff who are performing relatively routine, repetitive tasks. At another level, the attempt is to improve the quality of care, either by direct control or by providing the attending staff with an improved insight into the patient's physiological state. In this area, one generally hopes to justify cost on the basis of added value. Most systems involve a mixture of both".

An important pioneer function in this field was fulfilled by Warner (1969). He developed (at this stage on two large mainframes) a versatile "computer-based monitoring system". Functions included in the system were the determination of derived variables, the detection of statistically significant changes, flexible display, data storage and retrieval and computer-based record-keeping.

In general, the investigators put their efforts into specific aspects of a system, such as: intelligent alarms (Shubin et al. 1971, Pluth et al. 1972, Lewis et al. 1972); closed loop control (Sheppard et al. 1975, Westenskow et al. 1983); decision making (Robiscek et al. 1977); hierarchical processing (Glaeser et al. 1975, Swoboda et al. 1976, Schillings et al. 1978); testing/monitoring of lung function (Gerbode 1973, Prakash et al. 1984a, Peters et al. 1985); fluid balance computations (Mikolajczuk 1974, Klovekorn et al. 1976); and in combination with database management (Wiener and Weil 1978).

Almost all investigators paid attention to the computation of derived variables and the generation of a record. Sheppard and Kouchoukos (1976) wrote a survey, covering the period up to 1976, about many of the investigations mentioned above.

About ten years after the start of these developments in intensive care, comparable developments in the OR began. Rampil and Flemming started with the development of a system for trend presentation (1978); Nandorff et al. (1980) showed the usefulness of automation for trend presentation in monitoring; Mitchell et al. (1979) and Blom et al. (1981) developed a system with on-line display and pattern recognition facilities and applied color in the next version (Meijler et al. 1982 and this chapter); Frazier et al. (1981) composed an extensive set of requirements for an "integrated anesthesia delivery/monitoring system with computer assisted record keeping" to be developed by them (in their development they gave priority to the automated anesthesia record and later to the coupling to the hospital information system already mentioned in Chapter 2); Hsiao et al. (1983) applied a color graphics monitor for waveform presentation; and Block et al. (1985) described their experiences acquired in the development and clinical use of two successive prototypes of computer-based anesthesia monitors. Again, most investigators put their efforts into specific aspects of a system: in man-machine interaction (Trispel et al. 1981); in on-line display (Demeester 1982); in monitoring of the EEG and/or its derivatives (Simons and Pronk 1983); in integration of EEG monitoring and hemodynamic monitoring (Pearlman and Gurman 1985); and in intelligent alarms (Ballast 1985, van der Aa and Feldman priv. comm. 1985). In many cases an automated anesthesia record is the main objective or is later added to a system (Chapter 7).

3.2 Configuration

Before continuing with the description of DADS a general remark with respect to its design must be made. DADS was designed to function as a research tool to assess to what extent automation in anesthesia is feasible and to what extent it is important. Thus it was not designed to replace the conventional front end equipment but to collect and process the information generated by it.

This means that the hardware of DADS was not chosen to enable sampling of waveforms with a high frequency content, such as PART and ECG, or to meet the requirements for electrical safety of front end equipment.

The configuration of DADS is shown in Fig. 3.3:
- A 16-bit LSI 11/03 microcomputer with a memory capacity of 64 Kbyte functions as the central processor for signal processing of up to 32 analogue signals as measured at the patient or at a device attached to the patient (e.g. ventilator) and for the coordination of system controlling.
- An analogue-to-digital converter for conversion of up to 32 channels with an accuracy of 12 bits per channel. The clock system of the LSI enables a sampling rate of 50 Hz per channel.

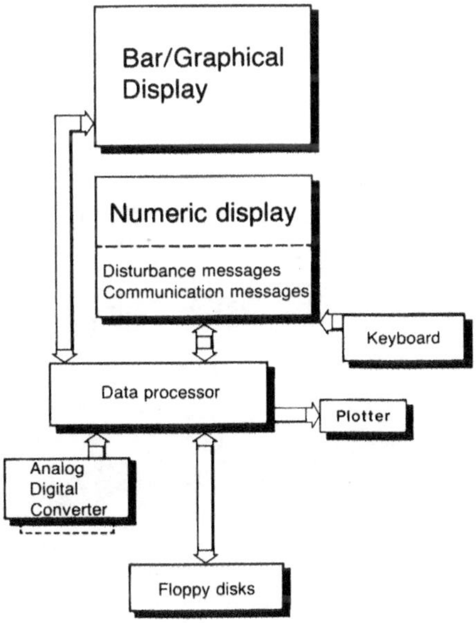

Fig. 3.3 DADS consists of a central data processor coupled to two intelligent display processors and peripherals for textual data entry (keyboard), data sampling (AD converter), data storage (floppies) and record keeping (plotter).

- The alphanumerical keyboard has an additional 25 function keys. The keyboard can be used to enter:
- commands to operate the system
- free comments and interventions regarding the course of the surgical procedure.

- Two display processors (Intel 8080) for the presentation of
- the measured signals and derived variables
- the man-machine interaction
- disturbance messages
- the system-generated user manual (HELP file)

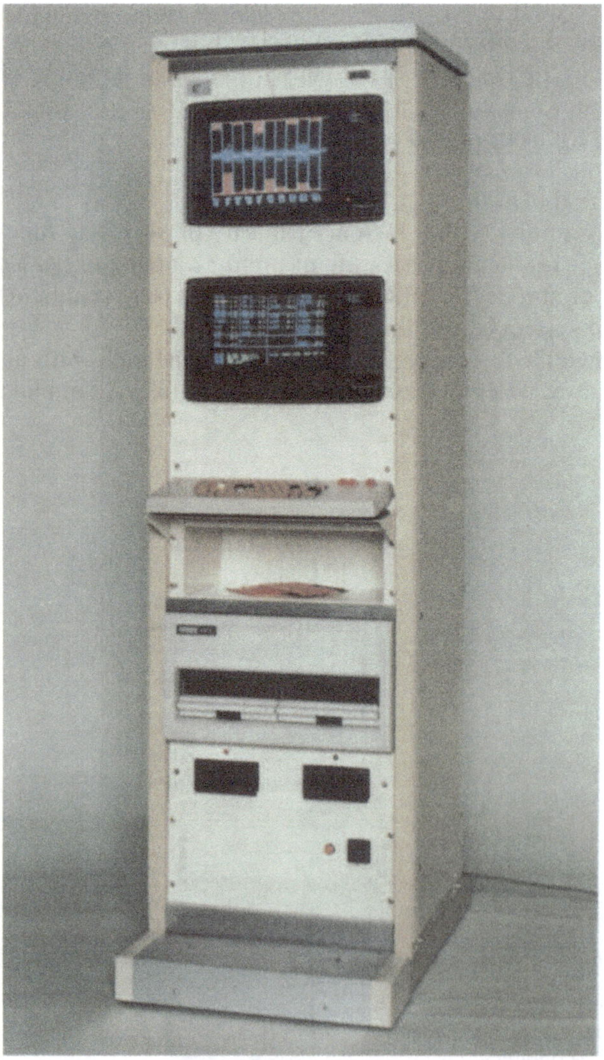

Fig. 3.4 The DADS system

- Each color monitor has a memory capacity of 32 Kbyte RAM.

Data presentation takes place by means of 8 colors and 32·64 characters or 128·128 pixels in the graphical mode.

- The two 8-inch disk units have a capacity of 512 Kbyte each for the storage of
- system programs
- 15 second values of the measured signals and derived variables
- disturbance messages
- entries via the keyboard

- A Philips PM 8151 plotter is incorporated for automatic generation of the anesthesia record.

Figure 3.4 presents a color picture of the DADS.

3.3 Data Flow and Processing (Disturbance Detection)

Two main flows of information can be discerned within the system: first, from the analogue-to-digital converter to the display processors and the floppy (Signal flow) and, second, from keyboard to processor(s) and floppy (Interaction flow).

Signal flow: After low pass filtering (40Hz), the measured signals are digitized in the AD converter and then sampled with 50 Hz (Fig. 3.5 a). In the central microcomputer the signals are processed in several stages (Fig. 3.6). An important result of the processing is that the system assigns a so-called state to each signal. All ac-

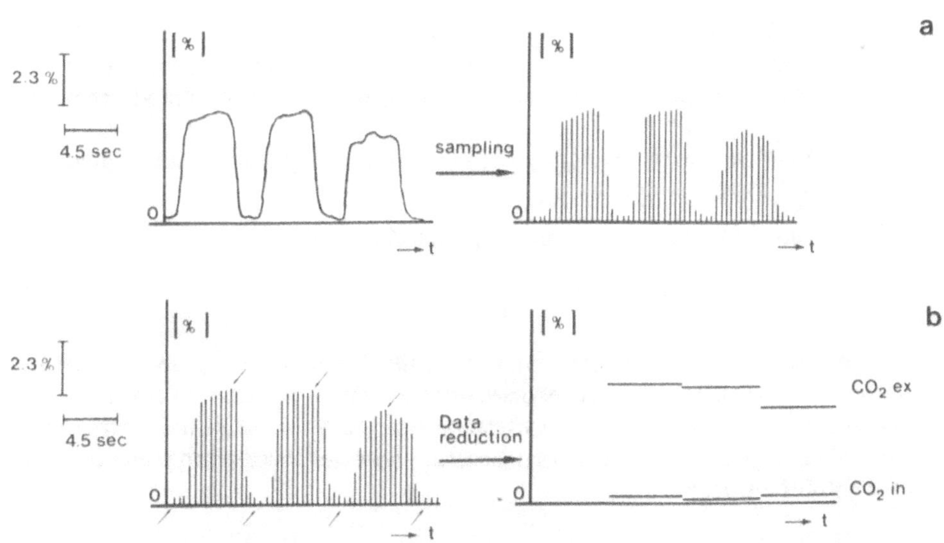

Fig. 3.5 The analogue waveform of (in this example) the percentage CO_2 concentration is sampled first **(a)** and data reduction takes place next **(b)**. Only the most relevant parameters are included in further processing.

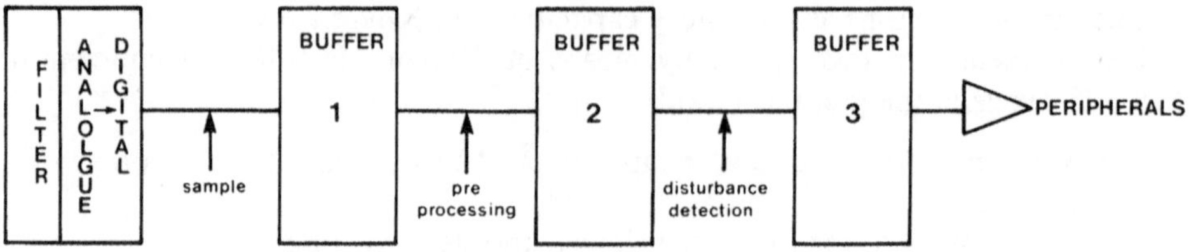

Fig. 3.6 The processing of the signals is done in several stages. Intermediate results are stored in buffers. Data which are disturbed by electrocautery are intercepted.

tions performed by the (pre)processing routines are determined by this state. The state is represented by a 4-bit code and is stored together with the 12-bit signal value.

Stage 1: The user indicates, by means of a command entered via the keyboard, that a signal is going to be used for monitoring. Thus a valid state is attached to that signal. (Otherwise the signal state remains invalid).

Stage 2: For all valid signals the sampled values are scaled to the range, as determined by their calibration settings. These calibration settings indicate which external voltage of the signal corresponds to the internal zero in the computer and which external voltage corresponds to the internal 4095 (2^{12}-1). If the new value exceeds the prescribed range the bad processing state is attached to it, and no further computations are performed on this value.

Stage 3: The electrocautery signal may disturb the measured signals in such a way that further processing is useless. Therefore, one of the 32 channels is reserved to indicate whether electrocautery is applied: at every processing stage this "flag" is checked. When it is set, no processing takes place until one second after stop of cautery; until that moment the last set of undisturbed data is presented to the user.

Stage 4: When no electrocautery is applied further processing takes place, depending on the type of signal.

Periodic signals: Maxima and minima are determined (Fig. 3.5b).

Nonperiodic signals: Additional filtering takes place in a 3.2-sec. low pass digital filter.

Ventilator phase signal: From one type of ventilator this signal can be obtained by means of a special interface. It recognizes three levels; the duration of each level indicates the inspiration time, the expiration time, and the pause time in the ventilation cycle respectively. In the preprocessing routines these parameters are computed from the phase signal.

The stages described above belong to the so-called preprocessing module. The resulting values, either direct signal values or derived values which together may amount to a maximum of 64 variables, are placed in buffer 2 together with their state. The buffer is updated every 100 ms for nonperiodic signals and at a new maximum or minimum for periodic signals. Once every second, the values from this buffer are subjected to a disturbance detection algorithm.

The Disturbance Detection Algorithm: Because so many variables have to be monitored, it is essential that DADS provides a higher level of data processing. To this end, more intelligent alarms have to be applied to provide the timely detection of clinically significant changes. In order to realize this a so-called disturbance detection algorithm was implemented (Appendix 3). This algorithm was developed to detect, in the first instance, statistically significant fast changes in the signals. As is standard practice in most conventional equipment, the algorithm first checks every variable to determine whether it exceeds its static alarm limits. These limits have been set by the user of the system and correspond to the limits as presented on one of the displays. When a limit is exceeded, the status "too high" or "too low" is attached to the variable. If the variable is within the static limits it is checked for dynamic disturbances.

The principle is that each new datapoint of a signal is compared to the signal's own behavior over the previous time period. This behavior is determined by the running average $\bar{x}_k$ over the last two minutes and the (running) mean deviation (d_k) over the last 15 minutes of each variable (update every second).

A dynamic disturbance is defined in terms of a new datapoint that exceeds its dynamic confidence interval of four times the deviation around the running average (Fig. 3.7). This means that alarms are generated only if the variable fluctuates strongly in comparison to its own previous behavior, since the confidence interval is self-adapting.

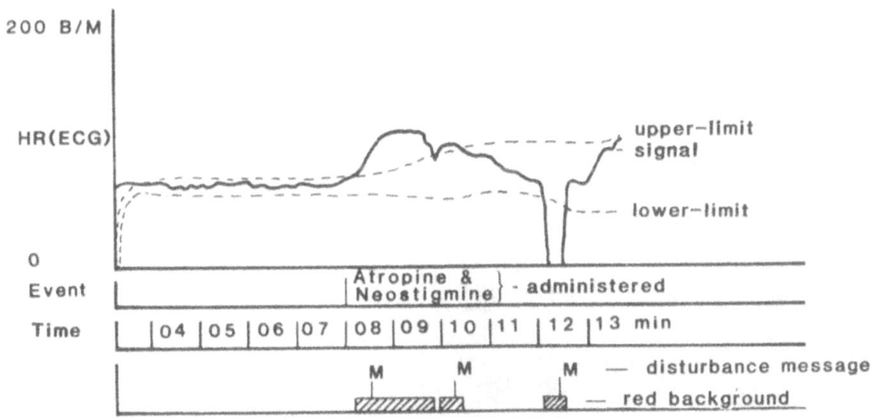

Fig. 3.7 The disturbance detection algorithm detects signal values outside an interval derived from the signal's own past fluctuations (mean deviation). In this example the confidence interval for the heart rate is shown (dotted line). After the heart rate has been declared valid it takes a short time before the confidence interval has been "learned" by the algorithm. Next, two disturbances and one artifact are detected. The user is warned of these occurrences by enhanced presentation of the signals on one of the system displays (colored background) and, when the disturbances are persistent, also by a message on that same display.

The algorithm performs an extra check on long-lasting deviations. At the moment when a confidence limit is exceeded, a counter is started which is incremented each time that the signal sample is beyond this limit and decremented when it comes within the limit. When the counter reaches 15, the disturbance is deemed persistent and an additional message is generated.

It must of course be questioned whether these statistically significant changes are also of clinical relevance. In order to answer this question the algorithm has been evaluated. The description of that evaluation can be found in Section 5.2.

Ultimately, the processing results in values of the variables which are updated every second in the last data buffer (no. 3, Fig. 3.6). Attached to these values are the ultimate states as generated during preprocessing and by the disturbance detection algorithm. The diagram of possible states which may result is presented in Fig. 3.8. The state of a variable will determine the way in which it is presented on a display.

Departing from this last buffer, messages with values of the variables and their states are sent to the various peripheral devices (Fig. 3.9). Every 15 seconds all valid variables, with their state, are copied to a buffer which, when full, is written to a floppy disk reserved for the patient data. (Another floppy disk is used for program storage).

Every 15 seconds a subset of 40 variables, together with their states, are sent to the upper color monitor for presentation in the so-called bar display. Every 7.5

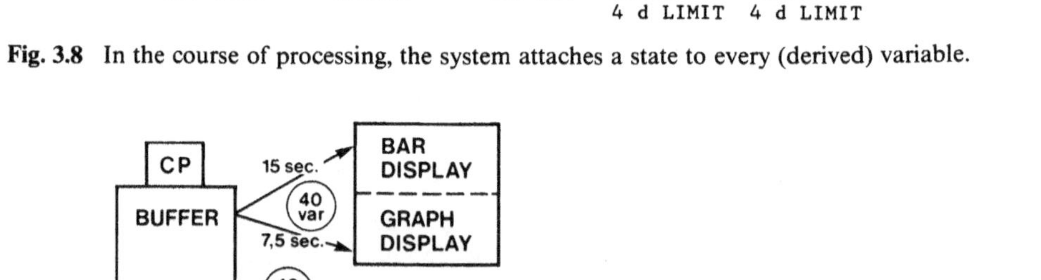

Fig. 3.8 In the course of processing, the system attaches a state to every (derived) variable.

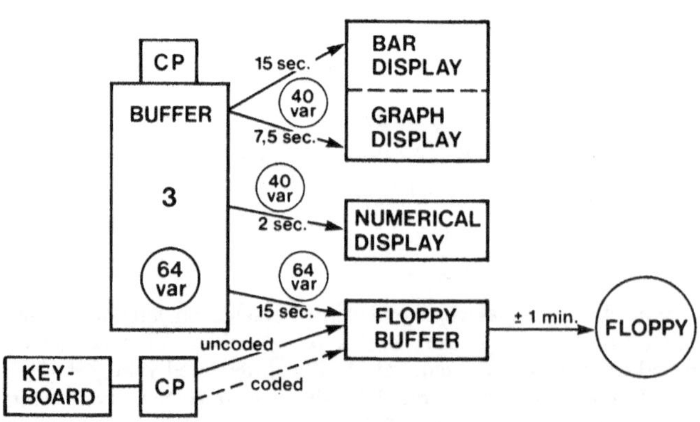

Fig. 3.9 Two main data flows in the system, from keyboard to floppy disk and from the AD-converter to floppy disk respectively, result in the presented and the stored information.

seconds this same subset is sent to the upper monitor for presentation in the so-called graphical display. (Bar display and graphical display may be exchanged on demand by the user). Every 2 seconds the subset is sent to the lower monitor for presentation in the numerical display.

Interaction Flow: The keyboard can be used to enter statements about the anesthetic procedure, for instance the administration of a drug, a surgical event, etc., and commands to handle the system, e.g. calling up another display format. The keyboard is attached to the lower display processor, in which an interpreter program has been implemented. This program takes care of the interaction between the user and the system. It checks whether a command is correct (syntax and semantics) and codes it accordingly. The coded messages are transferred to the central processor. There, depending on the code, the executable messages are used in a routine in the central processor or transferred to the display processor in question. All messages both executable and nonexecutable are sent to the buffer which is written to the floppy disk containing patient data.

3.4 Data Presentation

The problems with data presentation in the operating room having been recognized, the following requirements were imposed on DADS: DADS should enable centralized presentation of all (anesthesia related) data, when technically feasible (analogue signal available etc.), and should enhance pattern detection in the signals, for instance by means of trend graphs and comprehensive displays. To meet these requirements DADS was equipped with two display processors. These color monitors serve 4 purposes: man-machine interaction and presentation of HELP information, disturbance messages and patient data. Four different fields were defined on the color monitors (Fig. 3.10). Field 1 serves as a terminal which reproduces the interaction between the user and the system: the entered commands and the "answers" of the system are given.

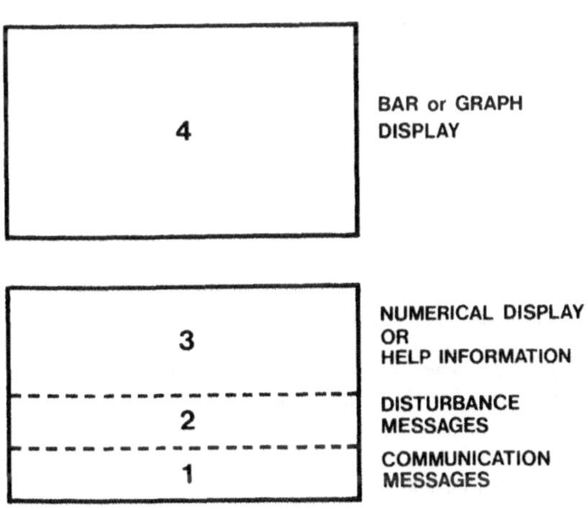

Fig. 3.10 The two color displays present the information divided over 4 fixed fields.

Because 6 lines are available, only the most recent interaction can be shown.

In field 2, five lines are available for the disturbance messages. All valid variables are checked against their static and dynamic limits (Section 3.3). When a limit is exceeded, this is internally represented by the state of the variable; externally, the presentation of the variable on the display(s) (fields 3,4) is altered.

For persistent changes, an additional message is generated in field 2. Other messages which are presented in this field include computer errors and messages indicating that a floppy disk is full with patient data or that a new sheet is required on the plotter.

The Numerical Display: The numerical display is usually presented in field 3. On this display, names and momentary values of up to 40 variables are presented. The 40 variables are divided over 4 columns and 10 rows. Separation lines can be placed in such a way that the variables can be grouped in functionally related blocks (Fig. 3.11). To avoid confusion it has been decided that regrouping of the information on this main overview display should not be accomplished during an operation. The state of the variable determines the colors in which variable name and value are presented (Table 3.1). Usually, the names are in blue and the values are in yellow on black.

Though the numerical display is visible most of the time, it can be replaced by a page of the "HELP file". When the user is learning to operate the system or is stuck when operating it, he can call for pages of this file (Section 3.5). Until the enter or return key is struck, the HELP information takes the place of the numerical display. (The messages with respect to persistent changes remain visible in field 2).

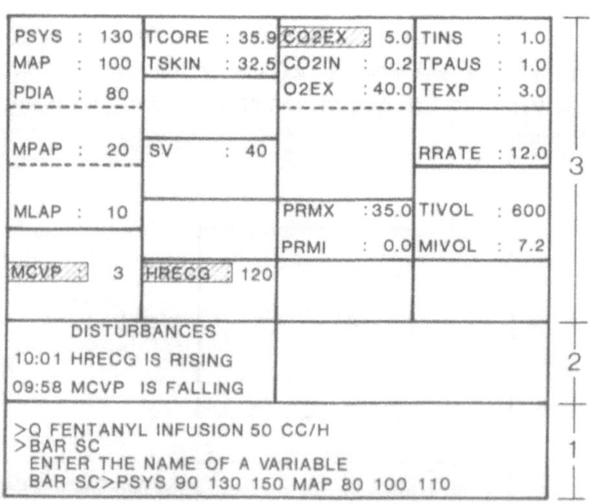

Fig. 3.11 The lower color monitor with the numerical display in field 3. Note the shading behind three variables indicating that the red background has been illuminated because a disturbance has been detected. Messages for persistent disturbances are given in field 2. An example of lines of interaction is presented in field 1. First a line with a quantitative comment, followed by lines with bar-edit interaction.

Table 3.1 The possible states, their meaning and the resulting colors of the variables on the numerical display.

State	Meaning	Message in field 2	Color of name in field 3	Color of value
0	invalid	-	no name shown	no value
1	input out of range	-	red on black	no value
4	dynamic alarm	fast rising	blue on red	yellow
5	idem	fast falling	blue on red	yellow
6	static alarm	above static limit	blue on red	yellow
7	idem	below static limit	blue on red	yellow
8	stable	-	blue on black	yellow
9	learning disturbance detection	-	blue on black	yellow
10	learning waveform detection	-	blue on black	no value

The numerical display is meant to provide the user with a centralized display of the momentary values of the variables instead of a display distributed all over the operating room.

In field 4, two display formats can be presented. One is the bar display, an alternative design (developed in collaboration with Ream) meant to stimulate pattern recognition. The other is a graphical display.

The Bar Display: The bar display is based upon the principle of the "artificial horizon". It provides the user at a glance with a global impression of the behavior of up to ten variables over the previous three hours. Each variable is represented in a bar graph. A bar is composed of five fields: two red alarm fields with (static) limits adjustable by the user (Section 3.3), two black attention fields and a central blue adjustable normal field (Fig. 3.12a).

The vertical scaling of a bar is linear. The normal value is always positioned in the middle of the screen. The alarm limit furthest apart from the norm value is placed at an extreme of the bar. The other alarm limit is positioned proportionally closer. The course of a variable is given by a small time plot (7 dots) on a logarithmic scale against the background of these five fields. The dot on the far right represents the most recent (present) value which is updated every 15 seconds. The second point from the left represents the average value over the previous interval (from 15 to 45 seconds ago). The next point to the left contains information over an interval which is three times the last interval (45 seconds to 2 1/4 minute), etc. The four right-hand dots thus represent information over the most recent 6 3/4 minutes. The update interval of 15 seconds, and thereby the range of the time plot, can be easily adjusted by the system programmer. Below the bar graph the name of the variable is presented together with the present value and the normal value, which are displayed numerically in "physiological" units.

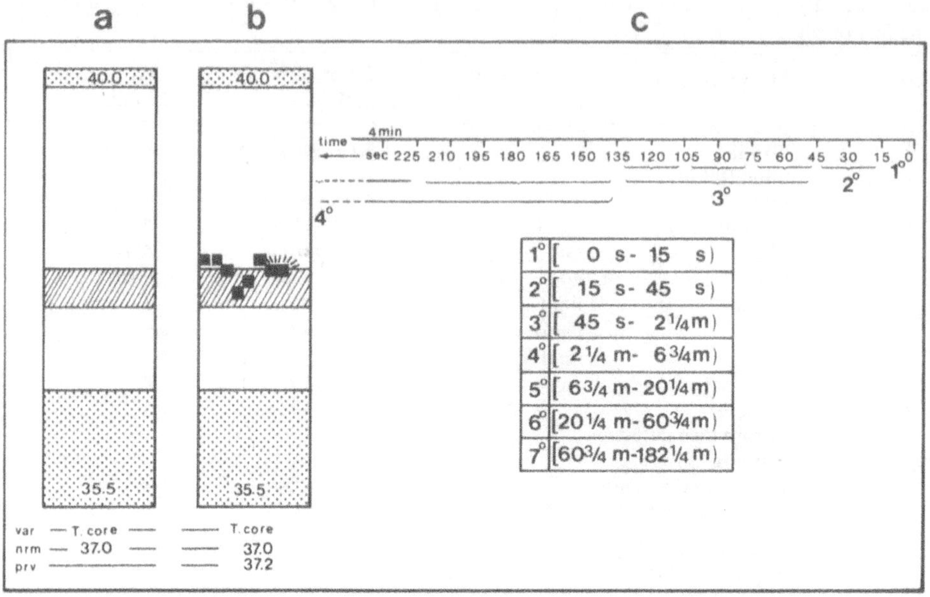

Fig. 3.12 In the bar display, for each of up to 10 variables at choice, one bar is reserved consisting of five fields including a central normal field and two alarm fields. Irrespective of the positioning of the alarm limits, the corresponding values are plotted at the extremes of the bars **(a).** As soon as a variable is included in monitoring (valid), its present value is transmitted every 15 seconds from the central processor to the memory of the bar display. In a condensed form these values are plotted as dots against the background of the five fields **(b).** Each dot to the left in a bar gives less detailed information regarding a period which is three times as long as the adjacent more recent period **(c).**

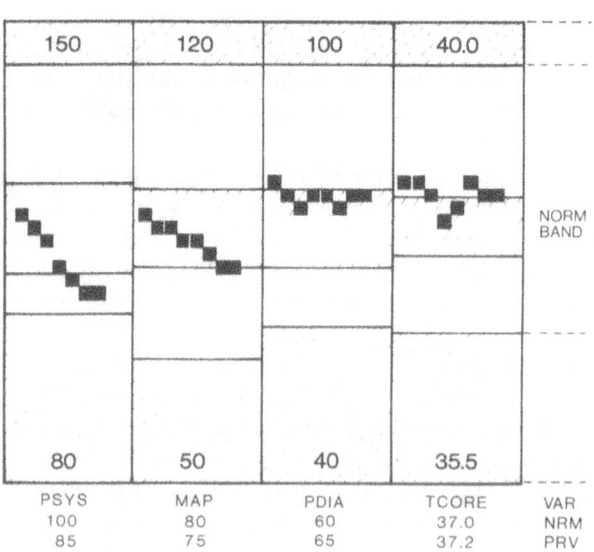

Fig. 3.13 Up to 10 variables may be represented by a bar in the bar display.

A proper selection of the ten variables represented in the bar display with their normal band and alarm limits, allows the user to make a quick assessment of the situation during anesthesia (Fig. 3.13). The following points can be considered:

- Is the situation normal, i.e. are all present values within the normal band?
- Is (was) the situation stable, i.e. are the dots at the far right, representing the recent history, within the normal band?
- Were there any large, long lasting changes in the past, i.e. are the dots representing the more distant history on a significantly different level than the dots on the far right?

On start-up, DADS presents a default bar display, but it is foreseen that in order to adjust the vertical scaling of the bars to the various phases of the procedure, on-line editing will take place.

The Graphical Display: The alternative presentation in field 4 is the graphical display. If information presented by the numeric and bar display does not give sufficient detail(s), the user can enter a command to compose or recall a graph.

In either one or two gratings up to four variables in each can be plotted on a linear time scale (Fig. 3.14). A choice can be made between 5 time scales: 15 or 30 minutes; 1, 2, or 4 hours. The momentary value of each plotted variable is given numerically at the rightmost pixel of the graph to which it corresponds. The vertical range of each variable is given in the upper left corner of the plot. It is possible to make the system generate coupled graphs (rods) for strongly correlated variables such as PSYS,MAP and PDIA which can be plotted together under the group name PART.

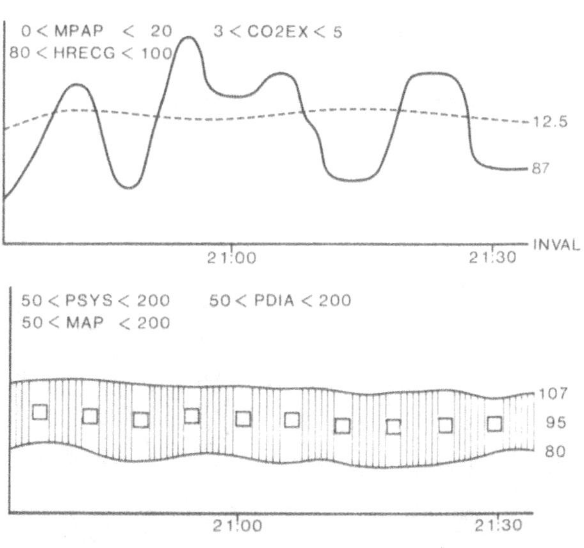

Fig. 3.14 A schematic example of a possible graphical display. This one presents three variables in the upper grating. Note: CO_2 has not been declared valid, thus no plot values are given. In the lower grating the group variable PART is drawn, which means that PSYS,MAP and PDIA are coupled by means of rods and they are plotted on the same scale (50 to 200).

By means of a single keystroke the default bar display and the default or last composed graphical display may be alternated. The default graphical display is preprogrammed but can be changed on-line. Moreover each user may compose (and edit) one additional graphical display. The benefit of the graphical display may be expected from the detection of slow trends which, using the equipment currently present in the operating room, are difficult to observe.

A final remark regarding the three displays: Because of the different updating frequencies the momentary value of a variable may differ slightly between the different displays. The update frequency of the numerical display is the highest and thus the values presented in this display are nearest to the exact present value. Because of limited memory capacity, this update frequency could not be used for the other displays.

3.5 Operation of the System

As mentioned before, operation of DADS takes place by means of a keyboard. The required interaction is minimal when DADS is only used for simple monitoring tasks. In that case it is sufficient to switch on the system and declare the specific signals valid. The numerical display is presented, and alternation of the bar and a graphical display is achieved by striking one function key. Thus, comprehensive monitoring is possible.

When, however, specific display layouts are required for specific applications, for instance for the bypass period, more (display edit) commands are required. If an automated anesthesia record is required as well, the various comments regarding the medical interventions must also be entered.

In order to enable efficient entry of commands and comments, a command set with a logical structure has been developed. Each command consists of a main command, possibly a subcommand, and a number of arguments or, in the case of comments, of a main command and text. To give the experienced user the means for accelerated entry of commands, various subcommands with their arguments may be entered in one command line.

Some examples of commands:

1	>BAR	SC	PSYS	80	112	130	ret
	on the bar display	the vertical scaling is changed	from the bar in which PSYS is shown	new low alarm value	new normal value	new high alarm value	dispatch command
2	>BAR	EB	8	NB	7	TCORE	ret
	on the bar display	a bar is erased	and that is the eighth	a new bar is made	to overwrite the bar at place 7	and TCORE will be shown	dispatch command

```
This is a command composed from:  > BAR EB 8
                                    and
                                  > BAR NB 7 TCORE
```

```
3          > C     START   BYPASS
             |               |
             a            followed
          comment          by free
                             text
```

In Table 3.2 a survey of the possible commands is given.

In order to minimize the number of keystrokes required for entry of the commands, function keys can be used. The keyboard is equipped with groups of function keys. One group is used to cover the most important main commands such as the show commands and the on and off commands. A second group includes all the signal groups which can be included in monitoring. In this way the second example requires 15 keystrokes instead of 21.

An experienced user can enter a composed command, but there are also facilities to help the inexperienced user. It is always permitted to dispatch an incom-

Table 3.2 The command set for operation of DADS.

BAR		bar display
BAR EB	[bar no]	erase
BAR EX	[bar no] [bar no]	exchange
BAR NB	[bar no] [var name]	make new
BAR SC	[var name] [low al/s**] [norm/s] [high al/s]	rescale
C	text	comment
CAL	[signal name]	calibration
GR		graphical display
GR 1	[var group name] [var names 1-4]	one grating
GR 2	U/L [var group name] L/U [var group name] [var names 1-4] [var names 1-4]	two gratings
GR T	[time axis 15/30/1/2/4]	rescale horizontal
GR SC	[var name] [low/s] [high/s]	rescale vertical
GR save		save as default
ON	[signal group names]	valid
OFF	[signal group names]	invalid
Q	text	quantitative data
SHOW		present
SHOW BAR		the bar display
SHOW GR L		the last graphical display
SHOW GR S		the default graphical display
STOP		stops DADS

** Instead of a new value the last default value may remain unchanged. This is indicated by entering the s (for standard).

plete command. The system comes back with a text in field 1 which explains to the user how to proceed with the command (in the examples below: user entry upper case, system reaction lower case).

Example: >GR 2 U ret
enter up to four variable names or
one group name followed by L
gr 2 u>PART ret (group name was entered)
enter L followed by up to four variable
names or one group name
gr 2 u part>L TCORE TSKIN ret (the command is
now complete)

Apart from this concise help from the system, it is also possible to call for the more extensive, system-generated user manual: the HELP file (Fig. 3.15). This is achieved by striking the special HELP function key. As a result, the numerical display is temporarily replaced by a page of the HELP file. The information presented in the page concerns the point in the command where the HELP was called for and refers to the possible (sub)commands or arguments with their meaning. The information is such that the system is virtually self-instructive.

In addition to these help facilities, there are also facilities to enable corrective measures in cases where an incorrect command is entered. When the user detects a mistake before a command has been dispatched, the whole command or part of it can be erased by means of either the erase line or the rub-out key. If there is a mistake in a dispatched command, this is detected by the interpreter program of the lower display processor. The faulty command is displayed again in field 1 with the first error in a different color. Additionally, as in the case of an incomplete command, the help line is printed. The user can then enter a corrective string. After dispatching this string, the interpreter program replaces the faulty part with the new string. Interpretation of the resulting command proceeds until a complete command is obtained or until a new error is detected.

Remark: at any moment during command entry it is permitted to cancel the command by hitting the ESCAPE key.

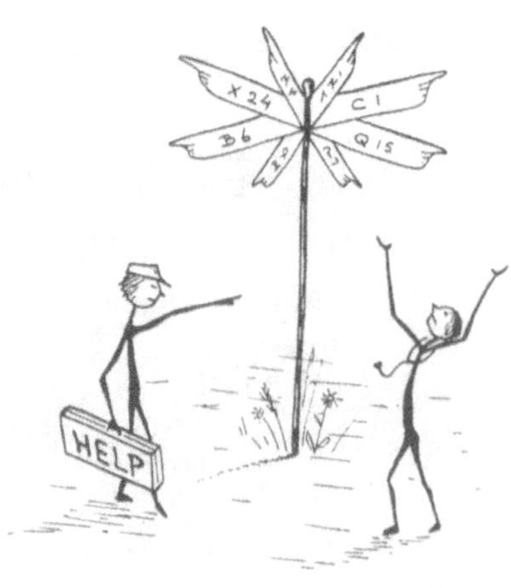

Fig. 3.15 The HELP file shows the user which way to go in the command paths.

Example 1:
a) >GR 1 PART CO_2EX T 4 ret
b) gr 1 part co_2ex t 4
c) enter time scale 15/30/1/2/4 and S if new standard wanted.
d) enter correction› ret
ad a) Note: both a groupname and a variable name
b) That is not allowed
c) System expects the time scale at this point in the command
d) CO_2ex is removed from the list by entry of an empty correction string and now the time scale is correctly the next argument.

Example 2:
a) >GR 1 PIRT T 4 ret
b) gr 1 pirt t 4
c) enter variable group name or up to four variable names followed by a time scale
d) enter correction› PART ret
ad a) A command with incorrect syntax of the group name
b) That is not recognized by the system
c) The system expects a correct name here
d) The argument is reentered correctly and replaces the incorrect string.

The Event Key: For a correct reflection of the course of anesthetic management, a synchronization of the medical interventions and the signal behavior is of utmost importance. Therefore it must be possible, with one keystroke, to indicate to the system the moment of such an intervention. To this end, an event key has been reserved on the keyboard. When this is hit, the time and serial number of the event are automatically stored by the system. Later, at a suitable moment, the anesthesiologist can enter the character of the event by means of a comment.

3.6 Data Storage

It is desirable in a research tool such as DADS to have both on-line and off-line access to the information regarding the course of the anesthetic procedure and the operation of the system. This is achieved by storing the keyboard entries and values of the measured and derived variables on floppy disk (Fig. 3.16).

First, all information is collected in the form of messages in the floppy buffer (512 byte). A message consists of a code as assigned by the interpreter, the (coded) contents of the message, and one additional byte to indicate the length of the message. Because the length of each message is known, the overhead required for stor-

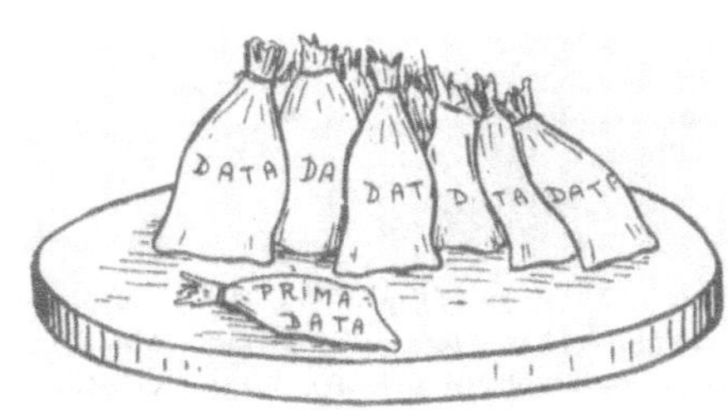

Fig. 3.16 The anesthetic procedure, including the operation of DADS, can be "replayed" because all data are stored.

age of the messages is minimal. At the same time the indicated length performs a pointer function to the beginning of the next message. A survey of all possible codes has been given by Zandbergen (1986).

The data messages are stored every 15 seconds, the remaining messages are stored on entry. The central processor couples a time message (code 60, length 3) to every stored message to provide the unique time - information relationship. One data message consists of 130 bytes. This means that it takes one minute to fill the floppy buffer which is then copied to the floppy disk. In this way floppy disk access noise can be kept to a minimum.

```
08:40:00   56   | 0  PSYS   8   112| 1   MAP    8   77| 2  PDIA   8   60|
                | 20   HR   8    67| 30 CO2EX   0   .0| 56 TCORE  7 15.0|
08:40:01   41   EVENT NR: 9
*******************

08:40:06   63   Q FENTANYL 2.5 MG I.V.
08:40:15   56   | 0  PSYS   8   117| 1   MAP    8   78| 2  PDIA   8   60|
                | 20   HR   8    66| 30 CO2EX   0   .0| 56 TCORE  7 15.0|
08:40:15   63   C 9 LARYNGOSCOPY
08:40:17   41   EVENT NR: 10
*******************

08:40:26   63   C   10  NTG.P. AAN
08:40:30   56   | 0  PSYS   8   110| 1   MAP    8   77| 2  PDIA   8   61|
                | 20   HR   8    64| 30 CO2EX   0   .0| 56 TCORE  7 15.0|
08:40:39   63   Q NTG P.   1UG/KG.MIN
08:40:45   56   | 0  PSYS   8   114| 1   MAP    8   77| 2  PDIA   8   61|
                | 20   HR   8    66| 30 CO2EX   0   .0| 56 TCORE  7 15.0|
08:40:58   63   Q ALFENT. 7.5MG I.V.
08:41:00   56   | 0  PSYS   8   111| 1   MAP    8   78| 2  PDIA   8   62|
                | 20   HR   8    67| 30 CO2EX   0   .0| 56 TCORE  7 15.0|
08:41:15   56   | 0  PSYS   8   115| 1   MAP    8   76| 2  PDIA   8   58|
                | 20   HR   8    65| 30 CO2EX   0   .0| 56 TCORE  7 15.0|
08:41:24   41   EVENT NR: 11
*******************

08:41:30   56   | 0  PSYS   8   112| 1   MAP    8   77| 2  PDIA   8   61|
                | 20   HR   8    67| 30 CO2EX   0   .0| 56 TCORE  7 15.0|
08:41:39   63   Q FENT.P.  .50UG/KG.MIN
08:41:45   56   | 0  PSYS   8   109| 1   MAP    8   73| 2  PDIA   8   59|
                | 20   HR   8    67| 30 CO2EX   0   .0| 56 TCORE  7 15.0|
08:41:52   63   C  11  INTUBATION
08:42:00   56   | 0  PSYS   8   111| 1   MAP    8   72| 2  PDIA   8   57|
                | 20   HR   8    68| 30 CO2EX   0   .0| 56 TCORE  7 15.0|
08:42:09   63   Q  ORBENIN 1G I.V
08:42:15   56   | 0  PSYS   8   111| 1   MAP    8   74| 2  PDIA   8   58|
                | 20   HR   8    70| 30 CO2EX   0   .0| 56 TCORE  7 15.0|
08:42:30   56   | 0  PSYS   8   110| 1   MAP    8   72| 2  PDIA   8   57|
                | 20   HR   8    70| 30 CO2EX   0   .0| 56 TCORE  7 15.0|
08:42:45   56   | 0  PSYS   8   111| 1   MAP    8   73| 2  PDIA   8   57|
                | 20   HR   8    68| 30 CO2EX   0   .0| 56 TCORE  7 15.0|
08:43:00   56   | 0  PSYS   8   111| 1   MAP    8   72| 2  PDIA   8   56|
                | 20   HR   8    68| 30 CO2EX   0   .0| 56 TCORE  7 15.0|
08:43:15   56   | 0  PSYS   8   110| 1   MAP    8   72| 2  PDIA   8   56|
                | 20   HR   8    68| 30 CO2EX   0   .0| 56 TCORE  7 15.0|
08:43:19   41   EVENT NR: 12
*******************

08:43:30   56   | 0  PSYS   8   116| 1   MAP    8   73| 2  PDIA   8   57|
                | 20   HR   8    69| 30 CO2EX   0   .0| 56 TCORE  7 15.0|
08:43:33   63   C 12 START RESCALING CONTROL VALUES
08:43:41   63   BAR  SC S 115 S
08:43:45   56   | 0  PSYS   8   114| 1   MAP    8   74| 2  PDIA   8   58|
                | 20   HR   8    70| 30 CO2EX   0   .0| 56 TCORE  7 15.0|
08:43:50   63   PSYS S
08:44:00   56   | 0  PSYS   8   112| 1   MAP    8   74| 2  PDIA   8   52|
```

Fig. 3.17 A sample from *REPORT*. Messages with the codes 56 (signal values), 63 (keyboard entry) and 41 (events) were selected. The occurrence of events is accentuated by a row of stars. In a later comment (command: C) the character of the event can be explained.

3.7 Off-Line Graph and Report Facilities

The data storage facility in DADS provides the possibility for off-line retrieval of data for all kinds of research. Two program packages for retrieval and presentation of data as stored by DADS have been realized. The first program, REPORT (Damman 1985) provides the user with the means to print out, chronologically and per patient, a selection of messages with a specific code and a selection of signals (with their state). Also, the time period over which the printout is desired can be selected. In this way for instance, man-machine interaction may be studied, all medical interventions can be printed out (C,Q codes) or signal behavior during certain interesting periods can be given in full numerical detail. This last option has been used for the study described in Chapter 5, where the correct marking of samples belonging to an artifact has been checked. In short, all possible combinations of messages over any time period of a procedure are retrievable (Fig. 3.17).

Numerical presentation of signal behavior may be required for certain specific applications but, in general, a graphic presentation will be needed. To this end, a graphical package was developed which consists of three programs: one program (TRGRAF) serves the transfer of the patient data from floppy disk to a file consisting of data messages only, which is also accessible for a PDP11 computer where the graphs have to be made; a second (SERIES) serves to create interactively a file with the layout specifications of the plots; and the third (GRAPH) creates the (color) plots.

A sample of a possible graph is given in Fig. 3.18. The possibilities for a graph layout are as follows: The time axis takes up the whole width of the paper (22 cm), but the time period plotted on this range may be chosen freely; the vertically available range is divided into five units; the vertical range for a plotted variable may

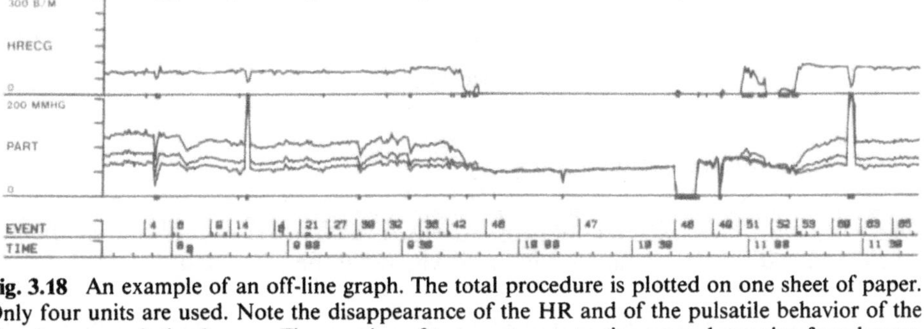

Fig. 3.18 An example of an off-line graph. The total procedure is plotted on one sheet of paper. Only four units are used. Note the disappearance of the HR and of the pulsatile behavior of the blood pressure during bypass. The crossing of temperatures at going on and weaning from bypass can be seen more clearly in the original colored version.

be chosen to consist of between one and five of these units; if, for a variable, more units are used, this of course reduces the number of gratings which can be plotted. The events are marked on a separate axis. The datapoints for which a disturbance was detected are indicated per variable (group) with tick marks.

3.8 Planned Facilities

For a short period, the final development phase of DADS and the first phase of the evaluation were concurrent. During this time some additional facilities of DADS were developed: some because they had already been planned and others because it followed from the evaluation that they would be required. Two rather essential facilities were implemented and tested but could not be integrated into the system because of its insufficient memory capacity.

For the sake of completeness we will mention these briefly.

The Numerical Display Editor: The bar and graphical displays can be edited on-line. For safety reasons this facility was not provided for the numerical display. However, it is desirable that the numerical display can be edited off-line to enable its adjustment to a different kind of anesthetic procedure or for special investigations etc. To this end the numerical display editor was developed (van de Lavoir 1984).

The Entry and Presentation of Noncontinuously Available Data: Until now only a relatively small number of signals have continuously been available in the form of analogue signals to be sampled by DADS. Other data, such as the adjustment of infusion pumps, administered drugs, blood gas values and electrolytes are only obtained intermittently as numerical values. The entry of these data in textual form following the C or Q command is, in fact, too cumbersome. To simplify entry of these data, a program based on ideas by Baetz et al. (1979) has been developed (Hees 1983). This program requires a greater number of function keys. Each group of data is placed in a menu which can be called up by means of its own function key. Depending on the character of the group, either the most frequently used item is the first on the list (as in the case of drugs) or the next item is presented at every call for the menu (as in the case of events). In this way a fast selection of the required item is ensured. The developed program has been adapted not only to enter the data but also to present them chronologically on a display which can be called up in place of the numerical display.

3.9 Concluding Remarks

In this chapter we described the properties of DADS as far as relevant for the user of DADS and for the evaluation aspects which will be discussed in the next chapters of this book.

The intricate details which had to be dealt with, and all the problems which were met during implementation of the programs, have not been mentioned. However, these may be of interest to people engaged in the development of comparable systems. Some of the important problems included:

- The communication between the different processors in DADS.
- The program for man-machine interaction in the lower display processor was originally written in BASIC to enhance flexibility and readability of the program. However, the BASIC interpreter was too slow to maintain an adequate interaction speed. The program had to be converted to machine language.
- An enormous amount of data had to be available to the upper color monitor to ensure prompt presentation of the bar or graphical display. Intricate tricks in data storage were required to fit all these data into its memory.
- The concurrency of all tasks to be performed by the central processor (sampling, computing, communication, interrupt handling) required a well-thought-out scheduling plan.

In the following chapters we will deal with the ergonomic and clinical aspects of the evaluation of DADS.

4 The Evaluation Method

4.1 Introduction

In this chapter we shall deal with a general evaluation method and with the one actually applied.

In *industrial engineering*, evaluation is a well-established method applied to many different situations. Its main application started out as the evaluation of jobs with the goal of minimizing production costs and maximizing interchangeability of workers, i.e. to increase efficiency (Moraal 1976). This led to task analysis and the procedures for finding the best workers for a particular task.

In *human engineering*, these techniques were extended to enable the design of optimal systems for automation of complicated tasks. Thus we used knowledge mainly from this field to derive the guidelines and foundations for constructing an evaluation method. We constructed the method in such a way that it is generally applicable to complex patient monitoring systems. The method covers the techniques as applied by several other investigators for the evaluation of complex systems.

Therefore, before describing the method we shall start with a short review of literature on the evaluation of complex medical monitoring systems.

4.2 Review of the Literature on Evaluation of Medical Equipment

Evaluation methods serve a dual purpose (Section 4.3). They have to provide both guidelines for improvements or redesign (evaluation of the situation for which a system is made) and tests to assess the impact of the system under study (evaluation of the performance of the system). In the literature we find papers which concern one or both of these aspects. Pace (1985) reviewed existing literature (MEDLINE) on the keywords anesthesia, monitoring and controlled clinical trials in order to find publications about the impact of monitoring systems during anesthesia on morbidity and/or mortality (outcome studies). Though he found a steadily increasing number of publications, of which 158 concerned all three keywords, none of these could be classified as an outcome study. Some of the publications described below may not meet stringent criteria regarding their statistical procedures but they come close to the classification "outcome study". Some other studies were performed by means of controlled clinical trials but measured the impact on other parameters, such as days in the ICU etc., rather than mortality/morbidity.

The first (as far as we could trace) publication concerning the evaluation of a complex monitoring system is by Pluth et al. (1972). It is a special publication because it concerns an objective study into the impact of a computerized intensive care unit in which data acquisition, storage, display, and decision making facilities are present. A population of 420 patients in the computerized intensive care unit was compared with 350 patients in standard intensive care. The factors which were checked for influence by the system are given in Table 4.1. Regrettably, there is no indication whether a statistical analysis was performed but still, according to Pluth: "these data suggest more prompt recognition and treatment of arrhythmias at an earlier stage in the computer unit, and the development of less serious arrhythmias and their sequelae such as cardiac arrest and death".

Bradshaw and Thompson (1975) were among the first who started a formal evaluation method with subjective criteria. The system under study was meant for collection, storage, and display of manually entered data, as obtained in a cardiothoracic unit.

By means of a questionnaire the views of the medical staff regarding user satisfaction and utilization aspects were collected. In addition to an overall positive reaction to the system, the staff mentioned a reduction in the access time to results: a decrease in telephone calls between operating theatres, laboratories, etc.; and an improvement in accuracy and quantity of information.

An objective evaluation with two components was performed by Hilberman et al. (1975). The evaluated system was used for calculation of variables which describe cardiac and pulmonary function at the bedside of critically ill patients, and served as a source for laboratory data. During the first years of its use a number of events which had previously caused "unexplained" serious arrhythmias or patient deaths were uncovered. In order to document such experiences, the investigators started a formal study of the effectiveness of the computer-based monitoring system in comparison to the standard monitoring system. The study consisted of two components: a study of the system's utilization by the clinical staff and a study of its impact on patient care. For the study of system utilization the type and character of user interactions with the system was recorded. The recorded information consisted of: time of interaction, user's job category, type of use (clinical or re-

Table 4.1 Factors included in the determination of the impact of a computerized intensive-care system (after Pluth et al. 1972).

Factor	Computerized	Standard
Duration of stay in unit (hr)	57	55
Vasopressor support (freq)	14.0%	14.0%
Antiarrhythmic drugs (freq)	24.0%	17.0%
Arrhythmia (freq)	0.7%	2.6%
Serious arrhythmias (freq)	20.1%	34.0%
Mortality rate (freq)	1.9%	3.4%

search) and the category of information extracted from the system. Alongside this, a statistical study was designed to investigate the impact of the patient monitoring system on morbidity and mortality in the ICU. For practical reasons, a strictly controlled clinical trial was not possible and a sequential study was performed. However they took care and also checked afterwards, that no significant differences in demographic data between the groups were present. Morbidity was estimated by days in the unit, days on a respirator and days with an arterial line. The cost aspect was taken into account and approximated on the basis of the morbidity measures and on the number of laboratory tests on blood gases. Although, among other things, the postsurgical mortality rate decreased from 9.3% to 7.7%, no significant differences were demonstrable (sample size 132 control and 207 new system) and the expected impact of the system could not be proven.

McClure et al. (1975) used a commercial computerized monitoring system and noticed that it was hardly ever used by the staff even after intensive training. Therefore they started afresh with an analysis of the problems regarding patient monitoring in the intensive care unit. They came up with valuable suggestions although the underlying facts are not given. They emphasized that the computer should be designed especially for those tasks suitable for it, e.g. automated record keeping. They also noticed the shortcomings of static alarms provided by a computer: computer alarms should be based on multiple data measurements, and artifacts should be excluded from the data on which alarms are to be generated. They pointed out that traditional criteria for measuring the quality of patient care (mortality, morbidity and length of ICU stay) are too excessive for judging the progress of a patient from a state of acute illness or distress to his ultimate state of health when discharged from the hospital or ICU. More subtle definitions of improved patient care have to be established. Some examples were given: elimination of mistakes in therapy, especially in drugs administration and in controlling fluid and electrolyte balances; reduction in the number of unusual events; and smoother progress of the patient towards recovery. To this end, they indicated the necessity of trend detection and prediction. Furthermore they suggested the use of the computer for the screening of chemical lab reports and for further education of ICU staffs.

Greenburg et al. (1975) realized the first objective analysis of information utilization in order to evaluate a computerized patient monitoring system. All keyboard requests to use the system were intercepted and stored so that frequency and sequence of access to the patient monitoring system could be determined.

Robicsek et al. (1977) performed a sequential statistical study to measure the impact of their all round system for computer-based intensive care. The system provided not only automated data collection, storage, and display but also an automated demand-regulated transfusion and infusion program and even a program for aiding in situation analysis and giving therapeutic recommendations. The ICU data of 400 patients who underwent open heart surgery just before the installation of the system were compared with those of an identical number of patients after installation. A significant reduction in the length of hospital stay in the new system group was found (15.2 ± 0.7 days to 13.8 ± 0.6 days, $p < 0.05$) and also a significant decrease in blood transfused ($1{,}600.8 \pm 127.5$ ml to $1{,}475.0 \pm 85.8$ ml, $p < 0.05$). A subjective but nevertheless definite impression was formed that patients connected to the computer had a much smoother recovery and their pressures and rates stabilized more rapidly and with fewer fluctuations than the conventionally managed group. Also, a 10 percent reduction in postoperative complications resulting primarily from respiratory problems was observed.

Bocquet et al. (1980) conducted a thorough study into the redesign of conventional anesthetic equipment. This study did not include automation but is a good example of methodical rearrangement and redesign and is applicable for computerized systems. The approach was as follows: they made up an inventory of comments on the conventional situation, illustrated with pictures, and the suggested modifications were listed. The anesthesiologist's working procedure was studied in detail and his work was separated into manual and visual activities. For each activity they determined:

1. Its duration
2. Its frequency
3. Its relative importance
4. Its relationship to other activities and anesthesia equipment.

A total of 15 procedures were videotaped. Manual activities were recorded by a single video unit with a wide-angle lens positioned behind the anesthesiologist's working area. Visual activities were recorded by means of an eye mark recorder. The activities were recorded from the film every half second. These data were entered into a computer file for sorting and statistical analysis. The results were used to draw sketches of possible arrangements of control, display and work surface. Full-sized cardboard mock-ups were produced of three possible systems; these were tested and subjected to the comments of anesthesiologists and manufacturers. A basic modular system was chosen and further attention was given to the control and display facilities and work areas. The resulting design became a slim unit occupying a small area, consisting of three vertically positioned modules and a permanently attached chart board. The lowest module was placed above the gas cylinders and housed the gas pressure gauges, the flow meter and vaporizer controls. The central module was the ventilator unit with the carbon dioxide absorber and an anesthetic circuit plus reservoir bag. The top module housed the ECG, the pulse monitor, and blood pressure gauge. The reservoir bag, being the most frequently checked visual display, was positioned close to the patient's head. The work area and storage cart were kept apart because they had little relationship to the control and display activities. The anesthesia delivery and monitoring system developed in this way is an example of well applied human engineering techniques. One other paper describes the use of filming techniques for advising on improvements in anesthesia equipment, though more globally (Drui et al. 1973).

A broad approach resulting in the design of a new integrated anesthesia delivery and monitoring system was followed by de Roo (1980). He performed a number of limited investigations into the task of the anesthesiologist during general procedures. The time spent on tasks and the time spent at certain positions was clocked, and the sequence of observations recorded. He determined the speed of the recorders required to enable detection of important patterns in various signals. Interviews were carried out to obtain remarks of the users regarding the conventional situation and opinions regarding properties of the new system. The concept design most favored by possible future users was a rack composed of a number of arrangeable units, with each unit containing one or more modules of the system. There was, as yet, no uniform opinion on the desirability of suspending the monitoring unit separately in a central position.

Galer and Yap (1980) developed two sequential prototypes for entering and storing of clinical intensive care data and compared these with each other and with the conventional situation. After concluding that the first thumbwheel prototype was unlikely to be acceptable, they followed a well-structured, five-stage program to obtain the next design: 1)feasibility and exploratory studies (limited); 2)developing the design concept; 3)construction and evaluation of a mock-up; 4)final specification and construction of a prototype; 5)evaluation of the prototype.

The new design was a keyboard unit with eight color-labeled groups of function keys and a numerical keypad set at an angle of 17.5^0 horizontally and a small display panel on top of this at an angle of 45^0 horizontally.

Evaluation included the time required for an entry and the proportion of entries transmitted which contained one or more undetected errors. For the twelve nurses participating in the evaluation it was shown that the keyboard unit produced significantly fewer errors than the thumbwheel unit ($p < 0.05$) and that the mean entry time for the keyboard was significantly less than that for the thumbwheel ($p < 0.001$).

In 1981, Collins et al. presented more general information on guidelines for evaluation, which did not provide additional insights.

A number of interesting evaluation studies have just been described. However, only Galer and Yap (1980) clearly mention having worked on both aspects of the evaluation: (re)design according to human engineering concepts and testing of the impact of the new design. As yet no complete general evaluation method for this kind of computerized monitoring system seems to exist. This is not suprising because the application of evaluation methods in medical systems is, in fact, at a rather early stage. In other applications such as in process industry, aviation and nuclear power plants (Hollnagel et al. 1983), much more effort has been put into human engineering.

4.3 Setup of the General Evaluation Method

Introduction: In this section we shall use literature on human engineering to compose a general evaluation method. The techniques and methods as used above are all elements of such a method. One advantage of departing from a general method, is that deliberate choices can be made regarding the practical realization.

Drenth (1976) describes a procedure which can be followed for the selection of workers. The term 'criterion' is introduced together with a 'dual procedure'. Potential workers are tested on their suitability for the task by checking on predictive criteria (requirements). Once they are settled in the job their proficiency is tested again, by checking on performance criteria. We find the same duality in procedures for the evaluation of technical devices. For instance, a new desk chair is being devised to diminish backache complaints. To this end, the seat is lengthened

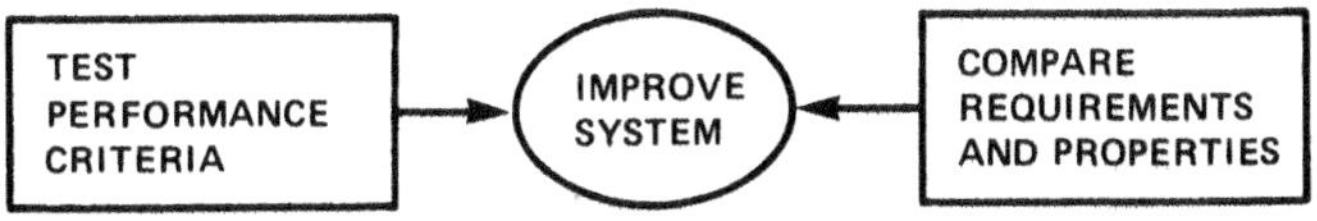
TEST
PERFORMANCE
CRITERIA
IMPROVE
SYSTEM
COMPARE
REQUIREMENTS
AND PROPERTIES

Fig. 4.1 In a complete evaluation method two aspects are treated: a test on the performance of the system (left) and a systematical check whether the system fulfills the requirements (right). Both stages may lead to improvements.

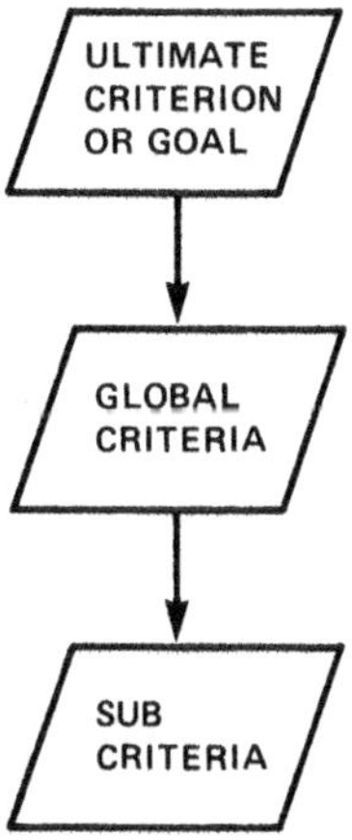
ULTIMATE
CRITERION
OR GOAL
GLOBAL
CRITERIA
SUB
CRITERIA

Fig. 4.2 The hierarchy in performance criteria. The subcriteria are the least excessive.

and the back and height are made adjustable. These are the (re)design criteria or requirements for the improved desk chair. However, to test whether indeed the chair does diminish complaints, tests on the performance criteria are necessary (Fig. 4.1), for instance on the amount of sickleave or more directly, complaints etc. From both aspects, suggestions for improvement can be derived.

For both "sides" of the evaluation the problem is to determine the criteria.

Performance Criteria: Regarding the determination of performance criteria Drenth (1976) gives some guidelines: Performance criteria have to be reliable, i.e. the test results should not be too much influenced by chance factors and the test must measure something in a fairly stable and consistent way. This can be enhanced by standardising testing conditions, making the test sufficiently long and selecting test items carefully. Performance criteria have to be relevant, i.e. they should be neither excessive nor deficient. "An excessive measure may cover part of the relevant properties while, at the same time, measuring additional phenomena which are not under control of the system" (Drenth 1976). A deficient measure is incomplete: relevant aspects of the performance of the system are left out. "Very often there is tension between reliability on the one hand and this aspect of relevance on the other. A final paper and pencil test at the end of pilot training provides a reliable criterion for selecting pilots. However, it is probably not as relevant as a test on their flying skills" (Drenth 1976). Finally, we must recognize that in most cases for a complete test more than one, mostly dependent, criteria have to be tested. We will distinguish three levels of concretization of performance criteria (Fig. 4.2).

The total aim of the process is called the "ultimate criterion" or "goal" (Drenth 1976). On this level we think of, for instance, "the total value of the company", "the wellbeing of the workers" which in monitoring terms can be translated to "improvement in patient care". Secondly, reference is made to "behavior or performance that is to be representative or indicative of the ultimate criterion, but in more operational and measurable terms". "Productivity per hour","quality of a piece of work" are examples of such concretizations (in monitoring criteria such as "mortality and morbidity" are probable). I will call them "global criteria". On a level which is still more concrete, Sanders (1976) gives examples of common performance criteria measures, which I call subcriteria (Table 4.2).

From these kinds of measure, so-called dependent criteria can be derived. For instance in order to test the new desk chair the dependent criterion "average duration of complaints over 20 workers, with and without use of the new chair" may be compared. Or, a more objective measure, the average tension in specific muscles may be used.

(Re)Design Criteria (Requirements): The other aspect of the evaluation process is the determination of the steps leading to improvement. This, in fact, is a kind of repeated and shortened designing process. To this end Bouma (1986 priv. comm.) uses a theory which prescribes that on the one hand, the model which the system to be (re)designed might have of the user must be determined, e.g. whether it is within the abilities of the user to operate the system by means of the 60 provided keys. On the other hand, the model of the system which the user forms should be

Table 4.2 Examples of subcriteria for performance testing of a person or system.

Subject	Examples
Time	reaction time search and inspection time movement time interresponse time total time
Action	accuracy (conversely errors) tracking movements aiming movements serial movements retention, recognition complex decisions psychophysical detection
Judgment	rating of importance rank order estimation of distances preferential choice
Physiological correlates	EEG cardiovascular responses muscle tension skin conductance respiratory responses

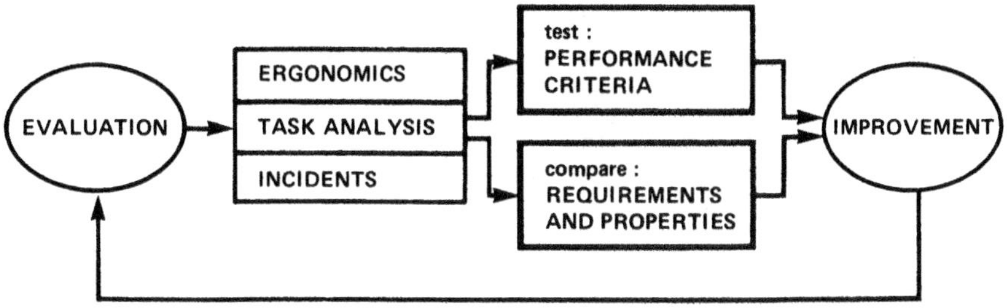

Fig. 4.3 In an evaluation method knowledge regarding three fields must be collected to derive performance and redesign criteria. The comparison between requirements and properties and the test on the performance of the system may lead to guidelines for improvements or to the decision that the system is ready for the next step in the design process.

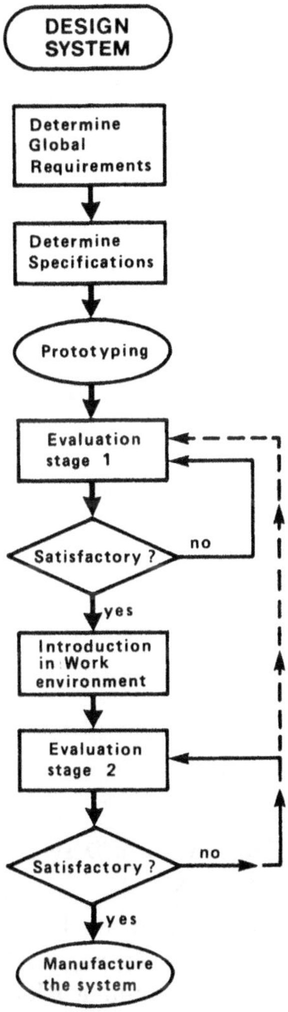

Fig. 4.4 A possible design sequence including two evaluation stages which are themselves iterative procedures as presented in Fig. 4.3.

determined, e.g. does the user expect the system to perform certain computations, or to be faultless? etc. Based on this theory a complete checklist for (re)design of a system can be composed (cf Section 6.1). Döring (1976a) gives also a set of (re)design guidelines. From these we extracted the conclusion that before redesigning can be done, knowledge on three basic subjects is essential: *task analysis, ergonomics* and *critical incidents.*

(Re)Design and Performance: Because both aspects of an evaluation may lead to improvements, it is the most plausible solution to use the same concepts from ergonomics, task analysis and critical incidents for the determination of the performance criteria. The following iterative scheme may then be used for an evaluation method (Fig. 4.3).

Information Retrieval: Above we gave guidelines for the generation of (re)design and performance criteria. The guidelines included the extraction of essential knowledge about the model the user has of the system under development. For this so called information retrieval, different techniques may be used, depending on the information we want to obtain. For instance, to specify new requirements for the desk chair, interviews with the personnel using the chair are useful but measurements of sitting posture may also give information. We have made an inventory of these different techniques (van der Stap 1982):

1 The interview of the individual by one or two (tandem) interviewers. The interview may be structured, open-ended, nonstructured, or nonstructured but focused.
2 The group interview; most common is the focused group interview
3 The questionnaire
4 Observations
5 Journal/ self-observation
6 The interview of informants
7 Unobtrusive methods ---
   ---> video recordings
   ---> audio recordings
   ---> signal recordings (physiological)
   ---> situation/environment tracing
   ---> literature study (archives,manuals, design specifications)
8 Simulation.

Evaluation and Design: In summary, a general evaluation method consists of the following:

Step 1- Apply the information extraction methods to obtain knowledge on ergonomics, task analysis and critical incidents.
Step 2- Determine a hierarchical set of performance criteria.

Step 3- Define sets of requirements by determining the model the user has himself formed of the system and of the model the system might have of the user. Include additional factors such as critical incidents and ease of maintenance.

Step 4- Execute the tests on performance and draw conclusions regarding the advantages and disadvantages of the system and the possible improvements.

Step 5- Compare the list of requirements with the properties and give suggestions regarding updating of the system.

Fig. 4.4 then presents a possible design sequence in which two evaluation phases are included.

4.4 Setup of the Evaluation Method as Applicable to DADS

In this section the general evaluation method will be adapted and elaborated in order to make it applicable to DADS. In the elaboration of Step 1 the justification will be given for the techniques which were applied as in Chapter 2 for obtaining knowledge on task analysis and ergonomics (of the operating room). In the description of Step 2 the considerations are given on which we based the selection of the performance criteria against which DADS was to be tested as in Chapter 5. The descriptions of the other Steps refer directly to later chapters.

Step 1 Step 1 of the general method prescribes the collection of knowledge on task analysis, ergonomics and critical incidents. In adapting this step for DADS, we selected the most suitable techniques for information extraction on the specific points about which we wanted to obtain information.

Task analysis: DADS influences the task and the working method of the anesthesiologists and possibly also of others in the OR because it is a monitoring system and thus might influence decision making. Besides, for optimal monitoring and data logging by DADS, the user has to enter the essential commands: this requires the attention of the anesthesiologist using the system and thus influences his actions. In order to obtain knowledge regarding the working method and task of the anesthesiologist without (and with) DADS throughout the total surgical procedure, the following possibilities were considered:

1) A literature study of task analysis and critical incidents:
   Performed and discussed in Sections 2.2, 2.4 and Chapter 8 respectively.
2) A video recording of (aspects of) anesthetics management, to be used for extraction of quantitative and/or qualitative information.
   Not performed. It was decided that even video cameras were too obtrusive and too elaborate to be applied in a situation were DADS was already an additional piece of equipment in the OR. Moreover, DADS could be used excellently as a recording instrument for all nonvisual inputs. However, we have some quantitative knowledge on workload because the literature study on task analysis was, among other things, based on two publications where quantitative knowledge was collected by means of video recordings (Fig. 2.7).

3) An activity chart for the registration of anesthetic interventions in order to obtain insight in the sequences of activities and the interrelations with surgical interventions and in type and frequency distribution of anesthetic interventions:

   An activity chart has been composed (Appendix 1) and discussed in Section 2.4.

4) Quantitative counts of type and frequency distribution of monitoring during anesthesia and of the character and frequency distribution of data logging:

   In the activity chart, the moments and type of intensive monitoring were pointed out. An inventory of the logged data is presented in Chapter 7 where the realization of an automated anesthesia record is treated. The time spent on tasks such as monitoring and data logging can be read from Fig. 2.7.

5) Mapping of the control function of the anesthesiologist:

   No quantitative study performed. However, global knowledge is applied in Section 6.4 where the layout of an integrated workstation is discussed.

6) Registration of critical incidents:

   Not performed systematically: too obtrusive an investigation requiring too many specific and elaborate procedures.

7) Objective study into system utilization (compare with Greenburg et al. (1975) and McClure et al. (1975) (see Section 4.2).

   This study has just started. A program to convert DADS files to a Database Management System in order that questions regarding utilization over a number of procedures can be posed, has been completed (Zandbergen 1986).

Ergonomics: DADS changes equipment layout and data presentation in the operating room. Therefore, to improve DADS and to determine its impact, knowledge about data presentation, equipment layout, and control is necessary. The following possibilities for obtaining information were considered:

1) Collecting the properties of comparable scientific and commercial systems from literature:

   A global inventory of comparable scientific systems is given in Section 3.1. Our knowledge regarding interesting properties of and developments in commercial systems was kept up to date but is not included because of the rapid changes in these systems.

2) The study and mapping of data presentation and layout of equipment in operating rooms:

   Performed and described in Sections 2.3 and 2.4 respectively.

Step 2 On the basis of the available information, we defined a hierarchical set of performance criteria (Fig. 4.5) (see also Krischer 1982).

As global criteria we defined:
- the work situation of the anesthesiologist in the OR, subdivided into work environment and workload
- the state of the patient subdivided into per- and postoperative state and expressed in mortality, morbidity and critical incidents.

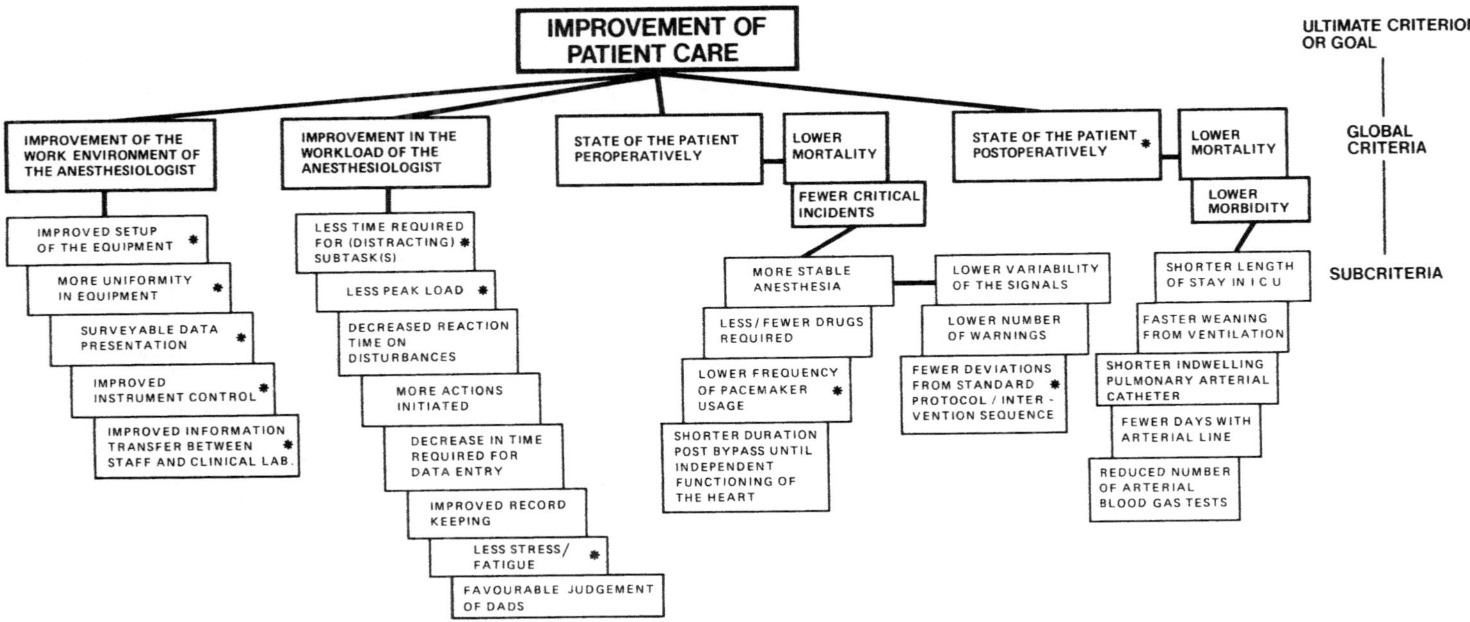

Fig. 4.5 The hierarchical set of performance criteria as applicable to DADS. For each of the subcriteria and some of the global criteria, tests can be developed to determine whether indeed the criterion is met with the application of DADS in the OR. For example, it can be tested whether fewer drugs are required during procedures with, as compared to procedures without, DADS.

It is clear that the list in Fig. 4.5 can be expanded with more criteria. Also, for a different system, another list would probably be composed. From this list the performance criteria to be subjected to testing can be selected: for instance, whether a decreased reaction time of the anesthesiologist on disturbances could be noted in procedures with DADS as against procedures without DADS.

The selection was based upon the following considerations:
- The sample size necessary for the test
- The measuring equipment available
- The correlation of the test with special properties of DADS
- The feasibility of the test based on some preliminary trials

Sample Size: Pace (1985) cites from a statistical source that, because of the low mortality rates, a sample size of 10,000 subjects would be necessary to show a reduction in mortality as the consequence of the use of a new drug or piece of equipment. To show a reduction in morbidity this number reduces to 450. To show a decrease in the occurrence of a specific critical incident something around this last number will also apply. When we make a selection from the more specific criteria lower in the hierarchy of Fig. 4.5, these will generally be less excessive, which reduces the required size of the test population.

Measuring Equipment: DADS is a powerful measuring instrument; it provides us with extensive means for data storage. As presented in Chapter 3, every 15 seconds all the continuously available physiological data are stored. The keyboard entries are stored immediately and placed in chronological order with the sampled data. The criteria in Fig. 4.5 were checked for their suitability for testing, with DADS used as the measuring instrument. As a result the criteria which are marked with an asterisk have not been included in further investigations. For instance, to be able to perform exact time measurements, video recording equipment is essential. Tests performed with this equipment are probably very useful but at the time installation of the equipment was considered too obtrusive. Moreover, this kind of equipment was not easily available to us. In principle, time measurements were believed feasible, yet we opted for the testing of criteria correlated with the group of physiological measurements which are collected and stored by DADS.

Special Properties of DADS: We stated previously that tests should be relevant: they should test especially those aspects of a system which are most obvious. The following aspects are the most obvious in DADS: 1) the algorithm for dynamic alarms with the corresponding change of the background color of the variable in question, 2) the bar display, 3) the trend display, 4) the automated anesthesia record, and 5) the data storage. The anesthesia record was developed as an element in the improvement phase (Step 3). The data storage is used as a measurement facility but has not yet been tested as to its impact on patient care. The efficacy of the red backgrounds and the bar display were chosen as the items to be subjected to testing.

The bar display was selected because of its relationship with the criterion "variability of the signals", and the red backgrounds were selected because of their relationship with the criterion "number of warnings".

Feasibility: Apart from the two tests mentioned above, some other criteria were thought to be relevant for testing. One of these was the "reduction of reaction time". However, this test did not appear to be feasible because only a limited number of disturbances was followed by an action with a clear onset (e.g. administration of a vasodilator as it follows a rise in blood pressure). The time delay between disturbance and action is so small that influences of DADS are very difficult to detect. Moreover, the operator could easily influence the accuracy of the method by inaccurate marking of the start of an action.

Though it is a global criterion, the criterion "critical incidents" seems to be very relevant. However, as a whole it is too excessive to be feasible. At a later stage it can perhaps be reduced to specific incidents which might be obviated by means of DADS and which then might be suitable as performance criteria.

Step 3 With respect to the redesign phase we tried to compose a list covering all requirements and properties of DADS. A sample part of the list which was composed by us is given in Section 6.1.

Step 4 The tests on the efficacy of DADS with regard to the number of warnings generated by the disturbance detection algorithm and the variability of the signals were performed and are described in Chapter 5.

Step 5 After a step-by-step comparison of the properties of the system with the requirements a number of minor improvements and some topics for major improvement were suggested and investigated. These include the topics to be described in Chapter 6:

- man-machine interaction (interaction facilities, interaction protocols and input devices)
- data presentation (legibility and the use of color)
- equipment layout (design of an integrated workstation).

4.5 Summary

In this chapter we gave a review of evaluation studies as performed on medical monitoring systems. Each of these studies covered only some of the elements for an evaluation study. Because no generally applicable evaluation method seemed to exist we tried to develop such a method ourselves. This method consists of two main components: the test of the performance of the system (test performance criteria) and the redesign of the system (determine redesign criteria). For the determination of the two kinds of criteria knowledge on task analysis, ergonomics, and critical incidents in the OR is a necessity. To acquire the required knowledge, a selection must be made from existing information retrieval techniques.

The performance criteria can be arranged according to a hierarchical structure from very excessive to rather specific. From these criteria a selection must be made determining which will be submitted to testing. For this selection some factors can be taken into account: the required sample size, the available measuring equipment, the correlation of the criterion with special properties of the system, and the feasibility of the test after some trials.

For the redesign phase it is advisable to check off all the facilities and missions of the system and in that way compose a detailed list of requirements. After a first overall check of the requirements against the properties, probably resulting in some minor improvements, a selection of some main subjects for systematic improvement can be made. In Chapter 5 the tests on two performance criteria are described, in Chapters 6 and 7 the major improvements are discussed, and in Chapter 8 the literature study on critical incidents is dealt with.

5 Evaluation: The Tests on Performance of DADS

5.1 General Introduction

In the previous chapter an evaluation method for computerized patient monitoring systems was composed. In this and following chapters this method will be applied to DADS. Here two tests on the performance of DADS will be described.

The first test concerns the investigation of the clinical significance of warnings as generated by the disturbance detection algorithm of DADS. The second test regards the stability/variability of patient signals: the behavior of these signals might be positively influenced by their enhanced presentation on the bar display. Both tests were performed with a special operator for DADS, to ensure that DADS was only used for monitoring and would not divert the attention of the anesthesiologists away from the patient, since they were not yet sufficiently accustomed to the operation of DADS.

5.2 Efficiency of Warnings

5.2.1 Introduction

In Section 4.4 we listed as one of the performance criteria the number of disturbances as detected by DADS. A disturbance is detected by the dynamic part of the disturbance detection algorithm (Section 3.3 and Appendix 3) which warns for observations outside the $4d_k$ confidence interval around the variable's running average. A warning for such a change is given by showing a red background on the numerical display behind the names of the variables in question.

The message which is meant to be conveyed to the user by this red background is that possibly a clinically significant event occurred or is pending. Significance in this context means that it is desirable for the anesthesiologist to recognize the situation and/or to intensify his monitoring and/or to change the management of the patient.

However, it is only possible to generate red backgrounds for the correct situations when we know the relationship between signal behavior and events. DADS was used to carry out a practical study into the identification and quantification of those situations for which a warning (or alarm) is useful.

In the introductory phase of DADS in the OR a study was undertaken in which an independent observer related the warnings to actions of the attending staff (Kragt 1982). The staff, including anesthesiologists, surgeons and pump technicians, were not able to observe the warnings and monitored by means of the standard equipment. This provided us with information about how the warnings correlate with clinically significant situations; in this way, a control population was also obtained to enable a later phase of the evaluation.

Apart from the statistically significant signal behavior as determined by the disturbance detection algorithm, we know that there are certainly a larger number of clinically significant changes, which however do not exceed the $4d_k$ confidence interval. During the study the observer collected some additional information to get an impression of the number of clinically significant situations which did not produce a warning on DADS.

5.2.2 Method and Materials

A sketch of the position of the observer and DADS with respect to the standard equipment and staff in the operating theatre is presented in Fig. 5.1.

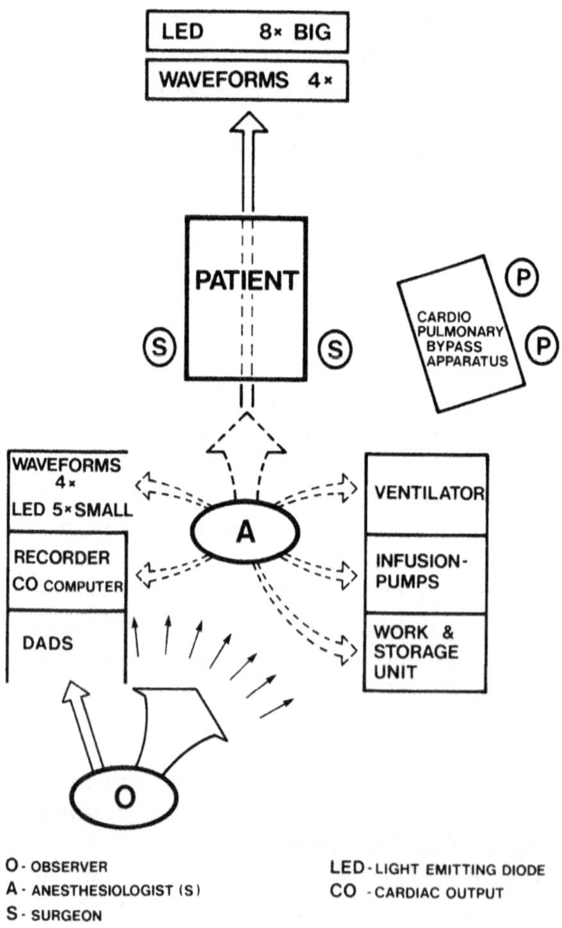

Fig. 5.1 An observer relates the warnings given by DADS with the actions of the staff. The variables to be monitored by the anesthesiologists are presented on the standard equipment by means of waveform displays, small and large LED displays for the digital values, and a set of miscellaneous displays on the ventilator and pumps.

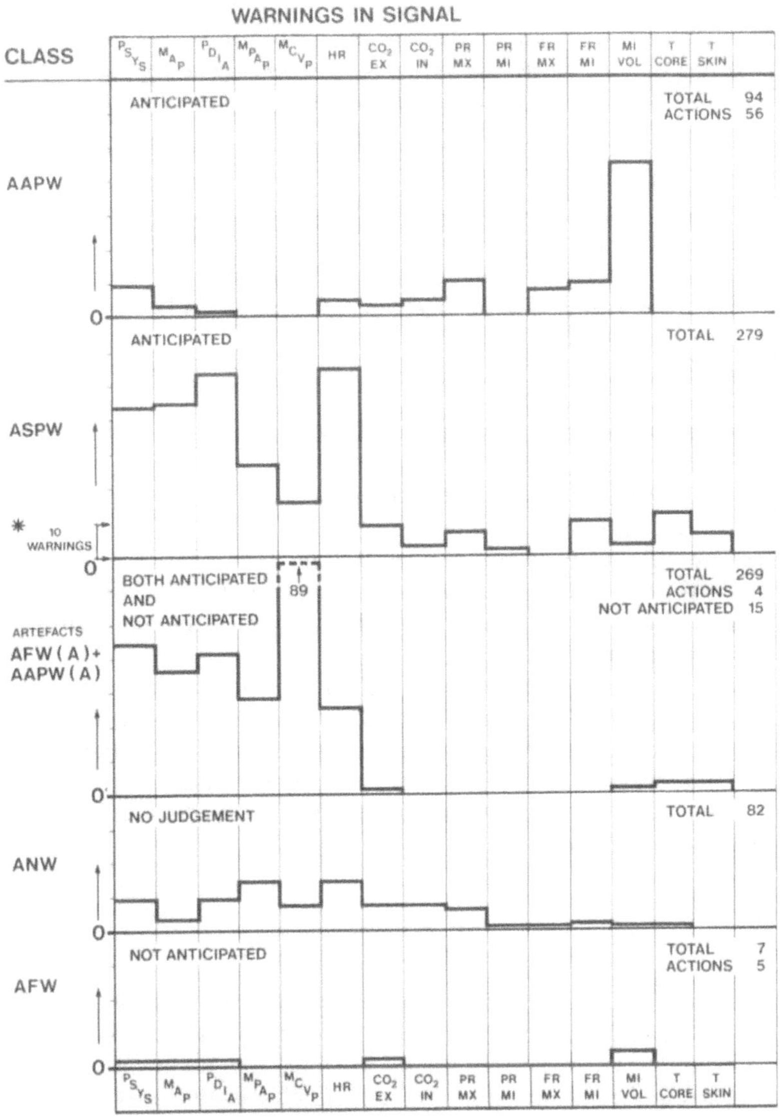

AAPW – ACTION OF ANESTHESIOLOGIST PRECEDED WARNING

ASPW – ACTION OF SURGEON (& PUMPTECHNICIAN) PRECEDED WARNING

ANW – ACTION COULD NOT BE RELATED TO WARNING

AFW – ACTION ANESTHESIOLOGIST FOLLOWED WARNING

A – ARTIFACT

Fig. 5.2 The warnings as generated by DADS were related to actions of the staff and classified. For each class the number of warnings per variable is plotted. Note: sometimes several warnings accompany one action. (* 1 unit = 10 warnings)

When a warning occurred, the observer used the keyboard to enter his observation of the actions undertaken by the staff around that moment. As explained in Chapter 3, these entries are immediately stored on floppy disk in chronological order with the data points and their status, which are stored every 15 seconds.

The relationships between warnings and actions were divided according to the following classification:

- AAPW - an Action of the Anesthesiologist Preceded the Warning: i.e. the warning is probably clinically less useful since the change was anticipated.
- ASPW - an Action of the Surgeon (or pump-technician) Preceded the Warning: i.e. the warning is probably clinically less useful since the change might have been anticipated.
- ANW - No Action could be related to the Warning; this could have three causes:

(1) The change was inadvertently missed by the staff and therefore not anticipated, so the warning might be useful.

(2) The change was anticipated but no action was necessary, so the warning might be less useful.

(3) The observer missed the related action.

- AFW - An Action of the Anesthesiologist Followed a Warning: i.e. the warning is clinically useful since the disturbance generating the warning might not have been anticipated.
- ARTIFACTS - Defined as disturbances with physiologically impossible behavior, such as 280 mmHg reached within seconds during flushing, or the disappearance of the waveform because of a pinched catheter.

These artifacts are considered to be a separate class because of their specific signal behavior. The corresponding warnings were either action-initiating (AFW) or quite useless (AAPW).

5.2.3 Results

During 6 cardiac surgery procedures the observer related 731 warnings as generated by DADS to actions of the attending staff. Fig. 5.2 shows the classified results.

The number of warnings for each variable is given per class. The total number of warnings can be read in the right upper corner, as well as the number of actions related to the warnings; there are fewer actions than warnings because sometimes a series of warnings was related to one action. In many cases such a series of warnings concerned several related variables, indicating a redundancy. To simplify the presentation of the results, 6 groups of related variables are distinguished:

RESP	Minute volume (MIVOL), maximal respiratory pressure (PRMX), minimal respiratory pressure (PRMI), maximal respiratory flow (FRMX), minimal respiratory flow (FRMI), CO_2ex, CO_2in
PART	Systolic arterial pressure (PSYS), mean arterial pressure (MAP), diastolic arterial pressure (PDIA)
TEMPS	Core temperature (Tcore), skin temperature (Tskin)

HR	Heart rate
MVCP	Mean central venous pressure
MPAP	Mean pulmonary arterial pressure

In the following, each class will be briefly discussed. If known, the character of the actions related to warnings for a group or a variable will be mentioned. In the case of the warning being caused by an action, this will be indicated as "group/variable disturbed by". For actions following a warning this will be indicated by "group/variable disturbed". In some cases, the apparent usefulness of the warnings deviated from the usefulness which was assumed above at the definition of the classes.

Class AAPW - 94 warnings (12.9%) were related to 56 preceding actions of the anesthesiologist:

Group/Variable	*Disturbed by*
PART	intubation and laryngoscopy→stress (probably useful after all) the effects of drugs (useful if reaction different from expected)
HR	---------------------------> stress (probably useful) external pacemaker switched on (less useful)
RESP	change of ventilator settings, about 5 times per operation and "big blow" (not useful)

Class ASPW - 279 warnings (38.2%) were related to preceding actions of surgeons and perfusionists:

Group/Variable	*Disturbed by*
PART	cannulation and change of flow CPB apparatus, smaller manipulations, lifting heart (probably less useful) sternotomy, cauterization, mediastinal dissection, pericardotomy, cannulation, closing mediastinum and skin -----------> stress (probably useful after all)
MPAP	manipulations of the surgeon (probably less useful)
MCVP	change of height cardiotomy apparatus and cannulation (probably less useful)
HR	manipulations of the heart by the surgeon (probably less useful), sternotomy, cauterization, mediastinal dissection, pericardotomy, cannulation, closing mediastinum and skin -----------> stress (probably useful after all)
RESP	manipulations by the surgeon (probably less useful)
TEMPS	covering patient with sterile drapes, cooling and warning up patient for CPB (probably less useful)

Class ARTIFACTS AAPW(A) - 254 warnings (34.7%) were related to preceding actions of the anesthesiologist:

Group/Variable	*Disturbed by*
PART	sampling and flushing (not useful)
MPAP	manipulation catheter or transducer (not useful)
MCVP	sampling, flushing, CO (not useful)
HR	derived from arterial waveform so also sampling and flushing (not useful)
RESP	disconnection of tube for sternotomy (not useful)

Class ARTIFACTS AFW(A) - 15 warnings (2.1%) initiated 4 actions:

Group/Variable	*Disturbed*
PART	resulting in cuff measurement (useful)
MPAP	resulting in change of catheter (useful)
TCORE	resulting in use of another temperature sensor (useful)
PART and HR	resulting in termination of pinching off catheter (useful)

Class ANW - 82 warnings (11.2%) could not be related to an action.

Class AFW - 7 warnings (1%) initiated 5 actions:

Group/Variable	*Disturbed*
PART	resulting in check of arterial line (useful)
MIVOL	resulting in switching the ventilation to manual (twice) (useful)
MIVOL	resulting in repair of a disconnection of the CO_2 measurement line (useful)
CO_2ex and blood gas	resulting in change of ventilator setting (useful)

5.2.4 Discussion

Observation of those actions of the anesthesiologists which were initiated by signal disturbances provided knowledge about clinically significant situations. In our investigation the range of disturbances exceeding an interval of $4 d_k$ around the running average was scanned. The proportional contribution of each class to the total amount of warnings is given in Fig. 5.3.

All 22 warnings in the classes AFW and AFW(A) were positively identified as useful. However, in other classes some useful warnings were also detected. By considering the number of warnings per class and per variable, and taking into account the level of usefulness which was stated on the basis of the corresponding actions, we estimated the following number of warnings as useful:

In the class AAPW actions such as intubation, induction, laryngoscopy and administration of (vasoactive) drugs may sometimes disturb PART and/or HR and/or MPAP in such a way that the generated warning is useful.

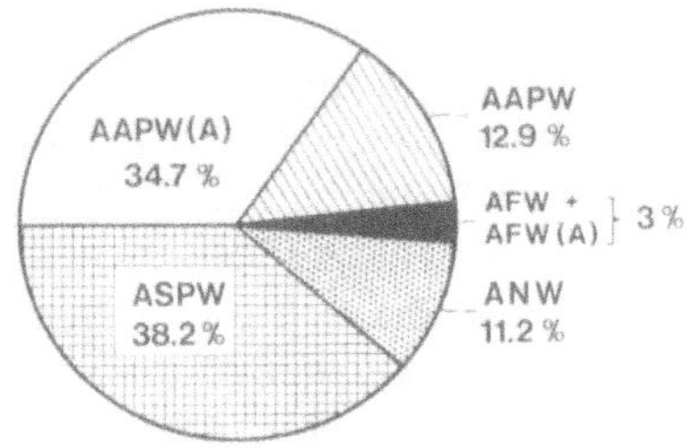

Fig. 5.3 The proportional contribution of each class to the total amount of warnings as generated during the 6 studies.

Action Followed Warning	AFW*	useful	3%
Action Followed Warning (Artifact)	AFW(A)*	useful	
Action Anesth. Preceded Warning	AAPW	useful	≃1%
Act. Anesth. Preceded Warning (Artif)	AAPW(A)	useless	
Act. Surgeon or Pump techn. Prec. Warn.	ASPW	useful	>3%
Action Not related to Warning	ANW	unknown	

* AFW+AFW(A)=3%

Assuming that, one action causes one disturbance in one-fourth of the studies and one-third of the variables, then we estimate the number of useful warnings in class AAPW at 8 (that is 1/12 of the warnings in this class).

In the class ASPW, actions such as cannulation, sternotomy, cauterization, pericardotomy, mediastinal dissection, and closing of mediastinum and skin may sometimes disturb one or more of the signals PART, HR, MCVP and MPAP in such a way that the generated warning is useful.

Assuming that, one action causes one disturbance in one-fourth of the studies and one-third of the variables, then we estimate the number of useful warnings in class ASPW at 23 (that is 1/12 of the warnings in this class).

For class ANW we only make the rough guess that no more than 50%, that is 40 warnings, might be useful.

Taking together the (possibly) useful warnings from AFW, AFW(A), ASPW, AAPW and ANW we come to an estimated total of 90 useful warnings, or 12% of the warnings in the 6 studies. When we exclude the 40 warnings in ANW we come to a total of 50: that is, 7% useful warnings.

The contribution to *useless* warnings is mainly caused by the definite artifacts, class AAPW(A) and by the manipulations of the surgeons which result in small artifacts in class ASPW. Because of their specific signal behavior it must be possible to realize an on-line detection and suppression of the artifacts in class AAPW(A). To this end a preliminary study was performed (Coolegem 1984) and an extension to the disturbance-detection algorithm is being developed. This is meant to suppress the artifacts in PART and HR as caused by flushing and sampling of the arterial line. It can be derived from Fig. 5.2 that in this manner about 120 (269-15-MPAP-MCVP-RESP) warnings can be suppressed and thereby the percentage of useful warnings increased to 8% - 15%.

Alcover et al. (1984) came to a comparable conclusion about how to deal with the contribution of artifacts to false alarms. They investigated computerized arrhythmia detection in the ICU during an 18-month period. The incidence of false-positive diagnoses ranged between 10 and 20 in 1000 beats. Movement artifacts accounted for 55.3% of all false-positive diagnoses, 0.8% of all interpreted beats were false negatives, and 3.8% were true positives. They stated that "artifacts often cause full-scale deflections with nonphysiologic amplitude and time constants. If analysis of these artifact's characteristics could be included in the computer algorithm, the incidence of false-positive diagnoses would be significantly decreased".

In principle, the test as described in this section can be performed with various thresholds ($n \cdot d_k$) for the generation of warnings and thus the inventory of clinically significant changes which was started above can be extended. However, we tried to get an impression of those clinically significant changes by observing the important actions *not* generating a warning. The following important changes were registered: about 5 slower changes (trends) and 5 changes in blood gas values, electrolytes and fluid balance management were observed to be action-initiating. For these, a warning would have been useful. The generation of warnings for these changes is also not without problems, however. Data which are not continuously available can as yet not be sampled by DADS (Sections 2.3, 6.2), and the generation of warnings on slow trends will probably increase the problem of superfluous warnings because the continuous stream of information and therewith the number of trends to be monitored by the anesthesiologist in the OR is enormous. Consequently the relative number of trends for which a warning is useful will be even smaller than in the case of the strong disturbances.

In conclusion: extensive research will be required before valid solutions are available which enable a system like DADS to warn exclusively for those changes which are clinically significant. At the moment we think that the solution might be found in the application of expert systems (Schoor 1986). In the knowledge base of such a system, specific properties of the signal behavior can be stored, e.g. regarding concurrent changes in the signals. It follows clearly from the test that changes in related variables often accompany the actions of the medical staff. If a red background is always shown behind each of a number of variables while their behavior is strongly correlated, a redundancy of warnings results. Raison et al. (1968) used this redundancy initially to lower the number of false warnings in their ICU. They studied the efficacy of alarms on the ECG and the pulse rate (from arterial pressure); during a 44 hours watch over eight days, ten patients passed through the two-bed station monitored by a single console. "A huge number" of 160 false ECG alarms and 173 false arterial pressure alarms was registered. They also watched over a period twice as long (21 patients), but this time only the coincidence of ECG and arterial pressure alarms was registered and only eight false alarms resulted.

The efficacy of warnings can also be considerably enhanced when the actions of the staff such as sternotomy, drug administration etc. are (automatically) known to the system. For instance, when the system has an electrical connection with an infusion pump it can detect the administration of vasoactive drugs and adjust its warning mechanism accordingly (of course, again on the basis of the knowledge) (Beneken and Gravenstein 1986).

In a study by Mitchell et al. (1983) into the usefulness of respiratory alarms in the ICU, the following important conclusions were made:

Useful alarms do not occur frequently. This is in agreement with our findings: per anesthetic procedure only about 12 of the 120 warnings were useful, which corresponds to 2 per hour.

In spite of, or rather because of, the low frequency of useful alarms, the computer-based system is effective. It provides a backup to remind the staff of the infrequent alarm states they fail to detect. Our opinion is that this conclusion is in agreement with the use of warnings by DADS: if a clinically significant situation remains undetected, it may give rise to a critical incident. During anesthesia the occurrence of such a critical incident is often not immediately recognized and sometimes only detected afterwards. Because the disturbances as detected by DADS are indicated immediately, it is likely that the detection of critical incidents might be improved. Therefore it is important to proceed with the optimization of disturbance detection algorithms until those critical incidents which may be prevented by an early warning in DADS can be recognized.

5.3 Controllability of Anesthesia

5.3.1 Introduction

In Section 3.4 we described the bar display of DADS. This display, based on the principle of the artificial horizon, enables the anesthesiologist to check at a glance whether ten of the most important signals are within an (adjustable) normal range. The concept of the bar display stems in fact from the following assumption: controlling the patient's signals within defined ranges is possible and is beneficial for the state of the patient.

At this point we shall describe a *pilot* study performed to obtain an impression of whether DADS with the bar display tends to influence the controllability of anesthesia. In Section 4.4 we mentioned that the number, duration and magnitude of disturbances can be used as possible performance criteria. These three performance criteria are, in fact, combined in the following controllability concept:

"The error of control in a variable is defined by the area between the signal and the normal range on the bar display during the time that the signal is outside this range".

5.3.2 Method

The starting point was to collect data from two populations: a control population (-D), where monitoring took place by means of the standard front-end equipment, and a population (+D) in which DADS could be used in addition to the standard front-end equipment. It was not possible to compare data from the control population with those obtained from a group exclusively monitored by means of DADS, because the front-end equipment could not be replaced by DADS (Section 3.2). Reasons for this were that, firstly, the signals have to be preprocessed by the front-end equipment before they are suitable for input into DADS and, secondly, at that stage of the investigation the anesthesiologists were not yet sufficiently acquainted with DADS to be able to do without the front-end equipment. For these reasons DADS could not be positioned closely enough to the patient to permit its exclusive use.

In the +D situation the bar display functioned as the main display. However it was permitted to exchange the bar display with a graphical display. The numerical display of DADS was kept at a fixed layout. In the -D situation the data displays of DADS were blanked. However, in both monitoring situations DADS was used as the unit for automatic registration of the patient signals and for recording of the data concerning the protocol of the study.

Apart from the quality of monitoring, there are, of course, other (more important) factors which influence the behavior of signals during anesthesia. These are: the patient, the type of operation, the anesthesiologist, the surgeons and probably many more factors.

Protocol: The following arrangements were made with regard to these main factors which influence controllability and therewith the character of the subpopulations included in the study.

The Anesthesiologist: Three anesthesiologists who were available were involved in the experiment: one was experienced both in cardioanesthetic procedures and with DADS; another reasonably so; and the third to only a limited extent. This added one degree of freedom to the study: not two subpopulations resulted from the study but six (Fig. 5.4a), i.e. three groups, each with half (5) of the studies with and the other half (5) without monitoring by DADS.

Type of Operation and Patient: The study population consisted of 30 patients, all subjected for the first time to coronary artery bypass surgery in the period from August 1984 to February 1985. The patients were premedicated with lorazepam and morphine. In all patients, an arterial catheter and a pulmonary arterial catheter were introduced. The anesthetic technique used was one of pancuronium and high dose fentanyl (and etomidate and/or alfentanil if necessary). The method of monitoring, with or without DADS, was randomly assigned to the patients included in the study. It was agreed that in some cases the patients would be excluded from the study according to the following:

- Inability to come from bypass without help (e.g. balloon pump)
- Unexpected occurrences during an operation necessitating an additional surgical intervention
- Intraoperative death
- Incompleteness of study measurements. The study continued until the required number of 30 patients was reached.

The Surgeons: During the bypass phase of a cardiac surgical procedure, signal behavior is primarily influenced by the surgeons and perfusionists. Therefore, this phase of the operation was excluded from the studies. Two time periods remained: first, from the start of induction to the start of bypass and second, from the end of bypass to closed skin.

Computed Surfaces: In Fig. 5.4b the surface areas which were chosen to be representative for the error of control are given. These surface areas will be computed

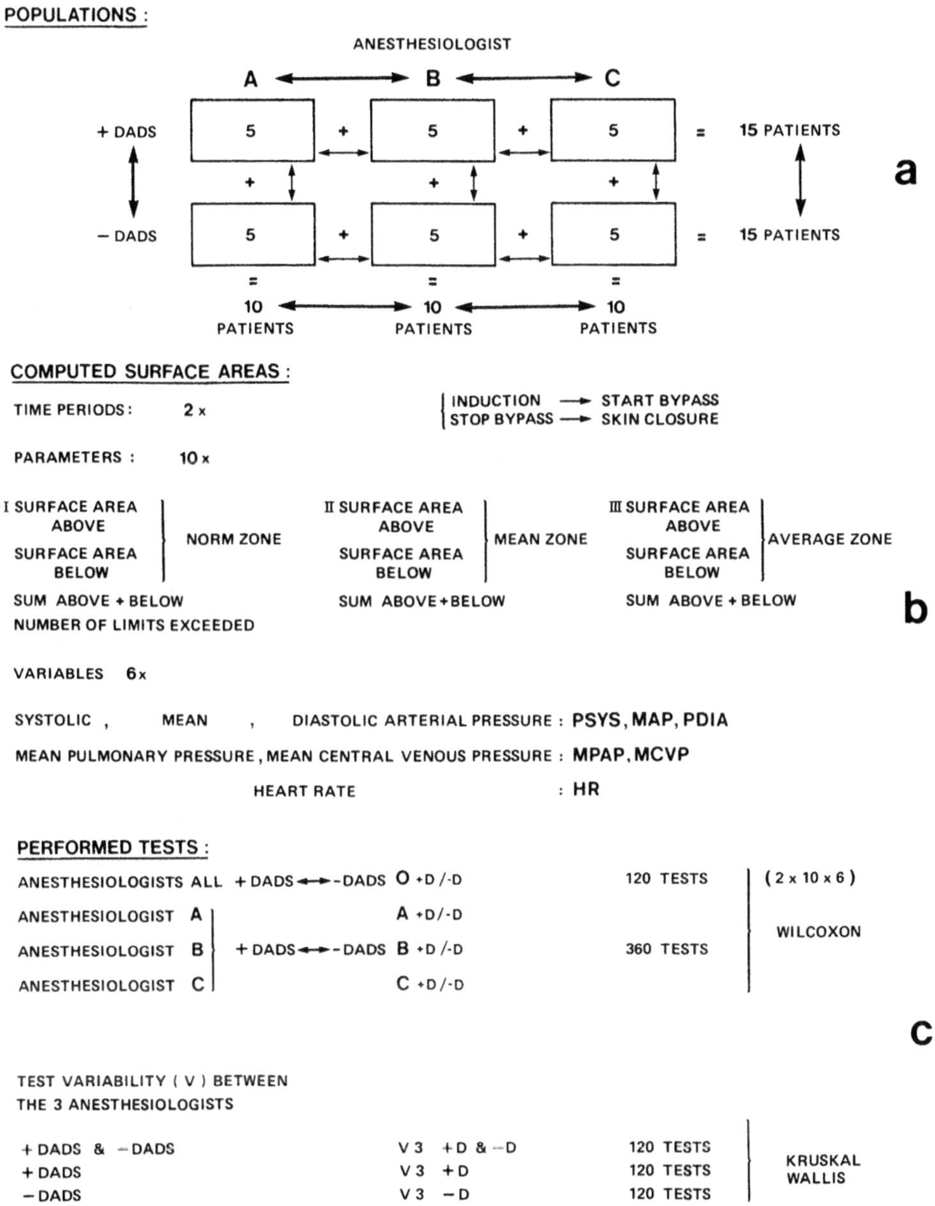

Fig. 5.4 This scheme indicates between which subpopulations tests were performed in the study (marked with arrows) (**a**), which controllability values were computed (**b**), and which tests were performed (**c**).

over several *time periods, variables,* and *parameters* and subjected to tests in order determine whether they are influenced by DADS as a monitoring system.

Time periods: The surface areas will be computed over the two time periods which have been mentioned above.

Variables: There is no agreement yet in the literature about the most essential set of signals/variables for monitoring during anesthesia. Depending on the type of patient some prefer hemodynamic parameters and others respiratory parameters. In our case, the participating anesthesiologists preferred hemodynamic variables, and a ventilator essential for automatic recording of respiratory signals by DADS was not available during the study. Thus we chose as the 6 control variables the systolic, mean and diastolic arterial pressures, the mean central venous pressure, the mean pulmonary arterial pressure and the heart rate. Together with "Tdelta", the difference between core and skin temperature, they constitute the 7 variables presented on the bar display during the study.

With regard to the width of the normal ranges, we could not find sufficient guidance in the literature although Berger et al. (1984) give some interesting indications. Therefore, we chose ranges of −15% to +15% around the selected absolute normal or target values of the variables. This was mainly based on our previous experience with normal fluctuations in arterial pressure and heart rate. Contrary to the description of the normal bands in Section 3.4, it was considered important for this study to give all the normal bands the same physical width on the screen in order to stress the horizon function of the bar display. The alarm limits were scaled accordingly.

The following rules of thumb were followed for the determination of the norm values to be used at the start of the first time period: norm values for PSYS, MAP and PDIA have to be chosen in such a way that adequate organ perfusion is warranted and norm values for MCVP and MPAP have to be based on preoperative catheterization values. If these were not available, norm values had to be chosen after placement of the pulmonary arterial catheter and before induction. The upper limit of the normal range of the MCVP is 15 mmHg. The norm value of the heart rate must be chosen in such a way that the lower limit of the normal range stays above 50 beats/min. In situations where it became evident that a signal could no longer be controlled within the planned normal range without detrimental effect for the patient, resetting of a norm value was allowed.

Parameters: There are, in principle, numerous ways to define and measure controllability. We may assume that anesthesiologists are using a kind of model when monitoring and controlling a patient. Knowledge about this model is our ultimate goal as this knowledge alone can lead to improvement in monitoring and control systems. Therefore, we defined the error of control in a number of different ways, each yielding specific information about signal behavior and thus possibly about the actual models used by anesthesiologists when monitoring and controlling a patient. The basic definition we chose for the error of control has already been given and is directly related to the method of data presentation on the bar display and thus (possibly) to the method of controlling applied by the anesthesiologists when they were using DADS.

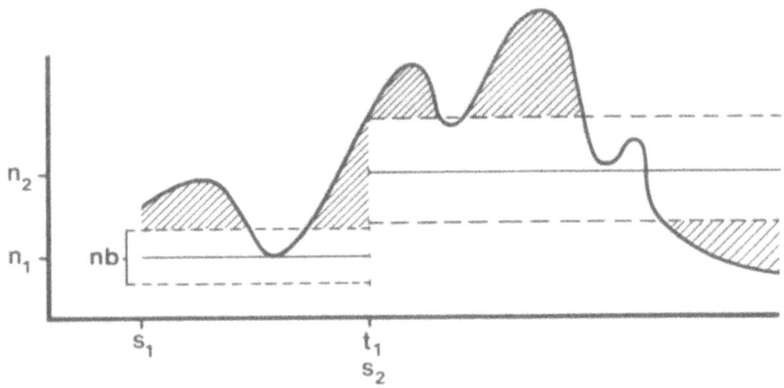

$$N = \sum_i \sum_{t \in I_i} (|x_t - n_i| - nb_i/2)^+ \Delta$$

where I_i is the set of sample points in

$$[s_i, t_i) \subset [t_b, t_e) \subset \text{surgical procedure}$$

and $a^+ = a$ if $a > 0$ and $= 0$ otherwise

$$nb_i = nh_i - n\ell_i \quad \text{with } nh_i = n_i + 0.15n_i$$

$$n\ell_i = n_i - 0.15n_i$$

Δ distance between two successive sample points

n_i the norm or control value as set by the anesthesiologist

Fig. 5.5a The first and original definition for the error of control: the surface area outside an adjustable normal (N) zone.

The following are the definitions we used for the error of control:

1. The surface area outside a zone of −15% to +15% around the (adjustable) normal zone (Fig. 5.5 a)

However, definition 1. does not take into account that the surface area may have been created with only a few strong fluctuations or with one very long but minor deviation of the norm zone. To include this aspect we used an additional parameter:

1a. The number of crossings minus one through the limits of the norm zone.

The values calculated according to definition 1, lack the following information: surface area that results from wrong settings of norm values while the signal behavior as such is rather stable without slow trends. This extra information is covered by the second definition for the error of control:

2. The surface area outside a zone of −15% to +15% around the mathematical mean of the variable (Fig. 5.5 b).

The difference in surface area, as calculated according to definitions 1. and 2. can be interpreted as a measure for the improper placement of the norm value.

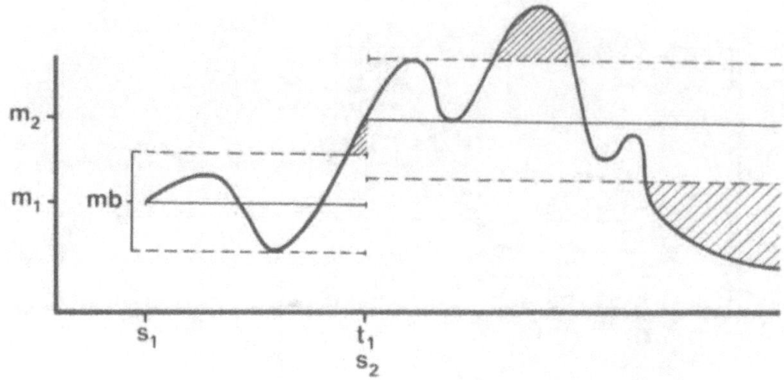

$$M = \sum_i \sum_{t \in I_i} (|x_t - m_i| - mb_i/2)^+ \Delta$$

where I_i is the set of sample points in

$[s_i, t_i) \subset [t_b, t_e) \subset$ surgical procedure

and $a^+ = a$ if $a > 0$ and $= 0$ otherwise

$mb_i = mh_i - m\ell_i$ with $mh_i = m_i + 0.15m_i$

$m\ell_i = m_i - 0.15m_i$

and $m_i = \frac{1}{k_i} \sum_{t \in I_i} x_t \Delta$ with k_i the number of sample points in I_i

Δ distance between the successive sample points

Fig. 5.5b The second definition used for the error of control. The surface area outside a zone around the mathematical mean (M).

Even so, the model on which the control actions of the anesthesiologists are based may not be completely described by these definitions.

A model can be envisaged where the anesthesiologists try to obviate fast changes but which adapts to slow trends, of course with the restriction that the actual values stay within reasonable limits. This is expressed by the third definition of the error of control:

3. The surface area outside a zone of −15% to +15% around the running average of a variable (Fig. 5.5c).

Apart from the total error of control the errors with respect to the upper and to the lower limit of the zones were also, separately, computed. Thus 10 controllability parameters resulted.

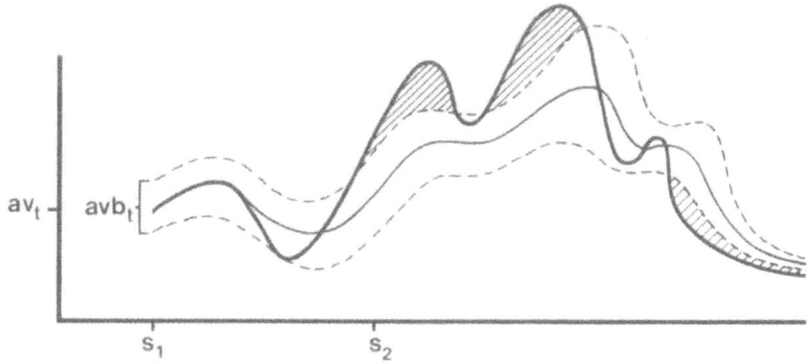

$$AV = \sum_{t \in t_b}^{t_e} (|x_t - av_t| - avb_t/2)^{+} \Delta$$

where $[t_b, t_e) \subset$ surgical procedure

and $a^+ = a$ if $a > 0$ and $= 0$ otherwise

$$avb_t = avh_t - av\ell_t \quad \text{with } avh_t = av_t + 0.15av_t$$

$$av\ell_t = av_t - 0.15av_t$$

and $av_t = av_{t-1} + (x_t - av_{t-1})/128$

Δ distance between the successive sample points.

Fig. 5.5c The third definition used for the error of control: the surface area outside a zone around the running average (AV).

Computations: For each patient included in the study, controllability was calculated over two time periods, for 6 variables and for ten parameters.

A special program, an extension of the *REPORT* program as mentioned in Section 3.7, was written for the off-line computation of the surface areas. In this program the DADS file is scanned twice. In the first run the data points belonging to an artifact (for definition see Section 5.2.2) are marked (see below) and the running average and mean deviation are updated with the 15-second data points, with exclusion of those which were marked as an artifact. In addition, the file is checked on the messages stating that one or more variables on the bar display have been rescaled. At these points, the zone around the normal and the mathematical mean over the previous interval with its corresponding zone are computed. With artifacts and mean zone determined, the 120 controllability values can be computed in the second run, in which the points marked as artifact are excluded. The importance of this measure is illustrated in Table 5.1.

In the first time period, 3 artifacts such as sampling of the arterial catheter corrupted the actual area calculation of 391 by a factor 3.5 to 1481. It is clear that this

Table 5.1 A sample of surfaces for study 2 as computed for PSYS with respect to the normal zone. In the lower part of the table the samples marked as artifact were not included in the surface computation.

VARIABLE	TIME PERIOD	INTERVAL (hours)	NUMBER OF SAMPLES	AREA AROUND NORMAL ZONE (mmHg. 15sec) above/below	
PSYS with artif.	T1	9.06.00-10.12.00	264	1388	93
				1388	93
	T2	12.39.00-12.51.15	49	0	1006
		12.51.15-13.07.55	67	54	12
		13.07.55-13.27.00	76	567	0
				621	1018
PSYS without artif.	T1	9.06.00-10.12.00	239	284	7
				284	7
	T2	12.39.00-12.51.15	49	0	1006
		12.51.15-13.07.55	48	20	12
		13.07.55-13.27.00	72	348	0
				368	1018

distortion of the values is unacceptable. To ensure the detection of most artifacts, DADS was equipped with a key for artifact-marking. At occurrence of an artifact, the operator of DADS pressed this key. In the program for surface area calculation a special algorithm was included to determine those data points around such a mark which belong to the artifact. Those points were excluded from surface area computations. This algorithm is described in Appendix 4.

Operator Tasks: As mentioned previously an operator for DADS formed part of the team and was responsible for the procedures related to this study; his tasks were the following:

- To enter the necessary commands to define or reset norm values
- To call up the graph display if the anesthesiologist preferred this for monitoring
- To enter on the keyboard data which are essential for a complete record of the surgical procedure but which are not automatically entered in DADS. These data are the administered pharmaca, the events, blood gas and electrolyte values
- To mark possible artifacts by means of the special artifact key. Occurrences for which an artifact mark had to be given included: Cardiac Output determination; manipulations of the table, transducers and catheters; sampling, flushing and drug administration through a measuring catheter. These artifacts are indicated by means of an asterisk in the event list of Appendix 2.

Finally, it is obvious that the operator had to maintain a neutral standpoint in that he had to refrain from actions and remarks which could influence the controllability study.

Performed Tests: The controllability values were compared by means of statistical tests.

Two hypotheses were tested:

H01: The display format with which the variables are presented has no influence on the error of control.
Because the material allowed it, the following subsidiary hypothesis was tested:

H02: The error of control does not depend on the attending anesthesiologist.
The statistical calculations were performed with programs from the SPSS package. The distributions followed by the controllability values are unknown and therefore non-parametric tests were used (Hollander and Wolfe 1973).

To test **H01** (two subpopulations, k=2) the (two-tailed) Mann-Whitney/Wilcoxon test was applied.

To test **H02** (three subpopulations, k=3) the Kruskal-Wallis test was used.

The performed tests are summarized in Fig. 5.4c.

5.3.3 Results

Controllability values were computed for the thirty patients. One patient was excluded from the study because a balloon-pump was used, and thus a supplementary study was performed. All patients but one had a medical history of myocardial infarction; 27 patients were kept on a maintenance dose of β-blockers, 17 had a maintenance dose of Ca antagonists, and 26 of nitrates.

Before the execution of the statistical tests, a check was performed to determine whether the dependent patient variables [e.g. New York Heart Association class (NYHA), duration of the procedure, extracorporal circulation (ECC) time, aorta clamping time, average age, blood pressure before induction] were equally distributed over the subpopulations, and thus did not bias the tests. In Table 5.2 the NYHA values and average age for the subpopulations are given. No significant differences occur. The same holds for the blood pressures before induction.

Table 5.3 presents the distribution of the mean length of the various time intervals over the subpopulations. In this table the ECC and aorta clamping times in the B +D group are significantly shorter than in the B -D group.

Another major bias on the tests may be the number of times the bars were rescaled in the O +D opposed to the O -D group. In spite of the rules which only permitted rescaling when the present norm value could not be maintained, the bar display is the main display in the O +D situation and thus rescaling might be more accurate (and therefore more frequent), causing a lower error of control,

Table 5.2 NYHA class and age distribution

POPULATION	NYHA class 1	2	3	4	AGE in yrs. mean	sd
A −D	0	2	3	0	53.6	10.5
B −D	0	0	4	1	53.0	10.8
C −D	0	1	3	1	59.2	10.5
A +D	1	1	0	3	56.0	10.2
B +D	0	1	3	1	57.8	8.4
C +D	0	2	1	2	62.6	6.0

Table 5.3 The mean length of the various time intervals which may influence controllability.

Population	Duration T1		Duration T2		ECC time		Aorta clamp time	
	mean	sd	mean	sd	mean	sd	mean	sd
A −D	71.8	6.4	55.0	7.5	118.4	30.7	62.8	22.2
B −D	74.0	18.8	58.0	12.2	144.8	31.7	79.2	15.2
C −D	75.8	16.3	49.2	7.4	108.2	31.6	53.8	14.1
A +D	74.4	6.4	53.0	10.5	131.4	44.3	68.2	28.4
B +D	83.4	21.1	57.2	17.6	79.2	24.4	42.2	19.5
C +D	64.6	10.7	51.6	11.7	134.8	30.1	69.4	15.5

though the quality of control is not necessarily better. The average frequency of rescaling was 7.9 ± 5.5 in the O -D group against 5.9 ± 15.2 in the O +D group, thus bias was not confirmed.

The main results of the performed tests are given in Fig. 5.6: for the Wilcoxon tests, the third column gives the number of significant outcomes in favor of DADS. In the last column the number of tests which showed a higher error of control with DADS are presented. For the Kruskal-Wallis tests the third column gives the number of times that a significant difference in error of control between the anesthesiologists was found. In this case the last column indicates the relative values of the error of control.

With respect to the two hypotheses the following conclusions can be drawn: When a great number of independent tests is performed, it is possible that by chance, a number of these tests have a low p value. Only when the number of significant p values exceeds 5% of the total number of tests (column 4) can it be stated that the outcome of the tests was significant. In this study, the parameters subjected to testing are not independent; thus this limit of at least 5% significant tests is probably even too low. This implies that only the V3 + D&-D tests give rise to a result which is probably significant. Thus:

H01: The display format with which the variables are presented was not shown to have a significant impact on the error of control.

H02: There is reason to presume that the attending anesthesiologist has a significant influence on the error of control.

Population	Total number of tests	Number p<0.05 in favour of DADS	Idem in% (critical value 5%)	Regards variables	In Time period	Remarks
WILCOXON O+D/-D	120	5	4.2%	MAP 1× HR 4×	2:5×	
A+D/-D	120	5	4.2%	MPAP 3× MCVP 1× HR 1×	2, 1:2× 1 2	MPAP T2 1× worse with DADS
B+D/-D	120	4	3.3%	MAP 1× PDIA 1× HR 2×	2 2 2	
C+D/-D	120	0				MPAP T2 5× HR T1 3× worse with DADS
KRUSKAL WALLIS V3+D&-D	120	Number of significant differences 10	8.3%	PSYS 2× MAP 2× PDIA 5× HR 1×	2 2 2 2	A rather low 4× B rather high 8× C rather low 2×
V3+D	120	3	2.5%	MPAP 2× HR 1×	1,2 2	A high 1× C high 2×
V3-D	120	5	4.2%	MAP 1× PDIA 3× HR 1×	2 2 2	A low 4× B high 5×

Fig. 5.6 The results of two statistical tests, performed to determine the impact of DADS (and anesthesiologist), on controllability of anesthesia are given. No significant influence of DADS on controllability could be demonstrated (Wilcoxon), but there is a possible significant difference between the anesthesiologists (Kruskal-Wallis).

Apart from these conclusions some interesting tendencies in the results can be pointed out:

1: Although controllability was not significantly better with DADS, it certainly was not worse. In the O + D/-D tests, 5 tests were in favor of DADS (column 3) with an average p value of 0.033 and 0 tests were worse with DADS (last column). When we consider the A,B and C tests we conclude that both A and B show a tendency to be positively influenced by DADS but that this positive result is nullified by C where 8 controllability values are significantly worse with DADS.

2: The improved controllability is, in most cases, found in the second time period. One reason for this may be that controllability is better after the heart has been "repaired". Another possible reason is that, in the first time period, the anesthesiologists learn to know the dynamics of the patient concerned (in terms of sensitivity for drugs, absolute signal values) and thus are better able to set the correct norm values and to control the signal behavior.

3: On average it seems from the V tests that the error of control for B is on a somewhat higher level than for A and C.

4: From V3 + D&-D and V3-D it follows that there is a difference in the controllability values of A and B. In V3 + D this difference has disappeared. From A + D/-D and B + D/-D we see that both show a tendency to do better with DADS. Thus we may conclude one of the following: DADS helps B more than

A so that they end up on the same level in V3 + D; B does more rescaling than A so that an artificially lower error of control is obtained; or controllability by B was influenced by yet another factor. The last statement is the most likely. We saw in Table 5.3 that for B the ECC and clamping times are significantly shorter with DADS. Under the assumption that these shorter times may reduce the error of control in time period 2, this might be the explanation of this result in the controllability tests.

In Figs. 5.7 to 5.10 the p value distributions for the N parameter group are plotted, both for the O + D/-D population and according to the anesthesiologists. For the O and the A tests the expected tendency towards improved control with DADS can be seen. For the B and C tests no shifts are present. Improved control by B with DADS occurred in the M and AV values (twice each). This is not so surprising when we know that the rescale frequency of B equals 12 as opposed to 4 for A and C. In this way the error of control according to definition 1. (N) for B was kept artificially at a certain level both with and without DADS.

5.3.4 Case Studies

In Section 5.3.5 we shall continue with a further discussion on the above results, dealing particularly with possible reasons for the low significance of the study outcome. Before this discussion, some samples of signal behavior with the corresponding error in control will be presented below. The samples were chosen on notable properties such as a high error of control with respect to the zone around the mathematical mean (M) versus a low value around the norm zone (N) etc. Apart from this, they are illustrative for all the possible combinations in surfaces around the norm, mean and average zones. To show a possible relation between signal behavior (and thus controllability) and medical interventions, those interventions which seemed to be of influence on signal behavior are also given. For studies 1, 2, 14 and 16 the graphs for two time periods and for study 20 the graph for the first time period are given.

Further comments on the samples are given in the legends.

5.3.5 Discussion

Above we dealt with the results regarding the influence of monitoring (and anesthesiologist) on the controllability of anesthesia as obtained in a pilot study consisting of 30 patients. No unambiguous significant results were found. The question is now: what are the possible reasons for the low significance? The low level of significance implies that DADS in its present form has no relevant impact on controllability. However, because of the positive tendencies which were apparent, it is more likely that there are other causes for the outcome of the tests. One possibility is that the time the anesthesiologists were able to spend on becoming acquainted with DADS was too short, so that they were not yet able to make optimal use of the new monitoring facilities provided by DADS. This may be partly

Fig. 5.7

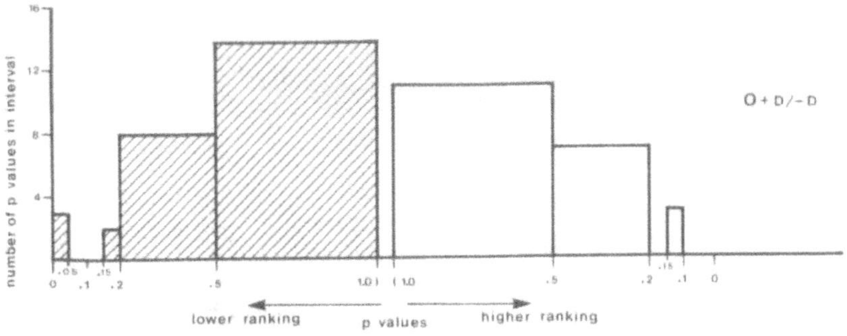

Fig. 5.8

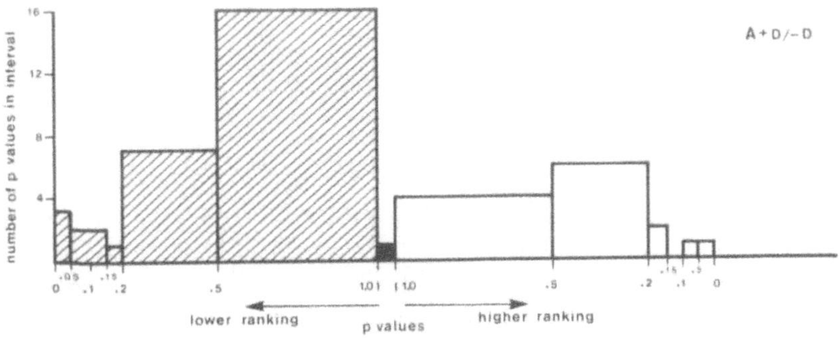

Fig. 5.9

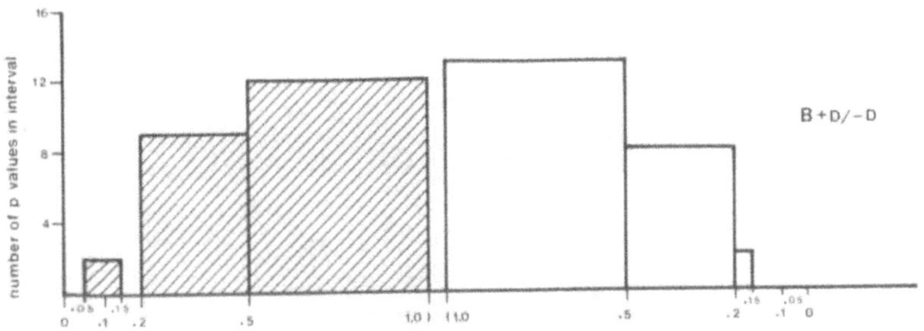

Fig. 5.10

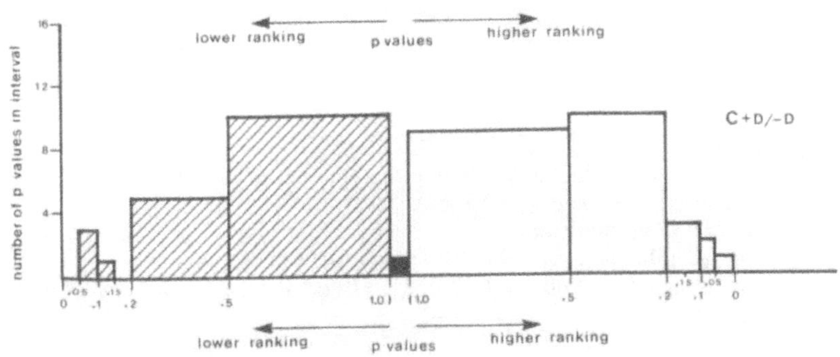

Figs. 5.7–5.10 The p value distributions for the outcomes of the Wilcoxon tests on the error of control according to definition 1 are given. Tendencies in favor of DADS can be seen in the O and A tests.

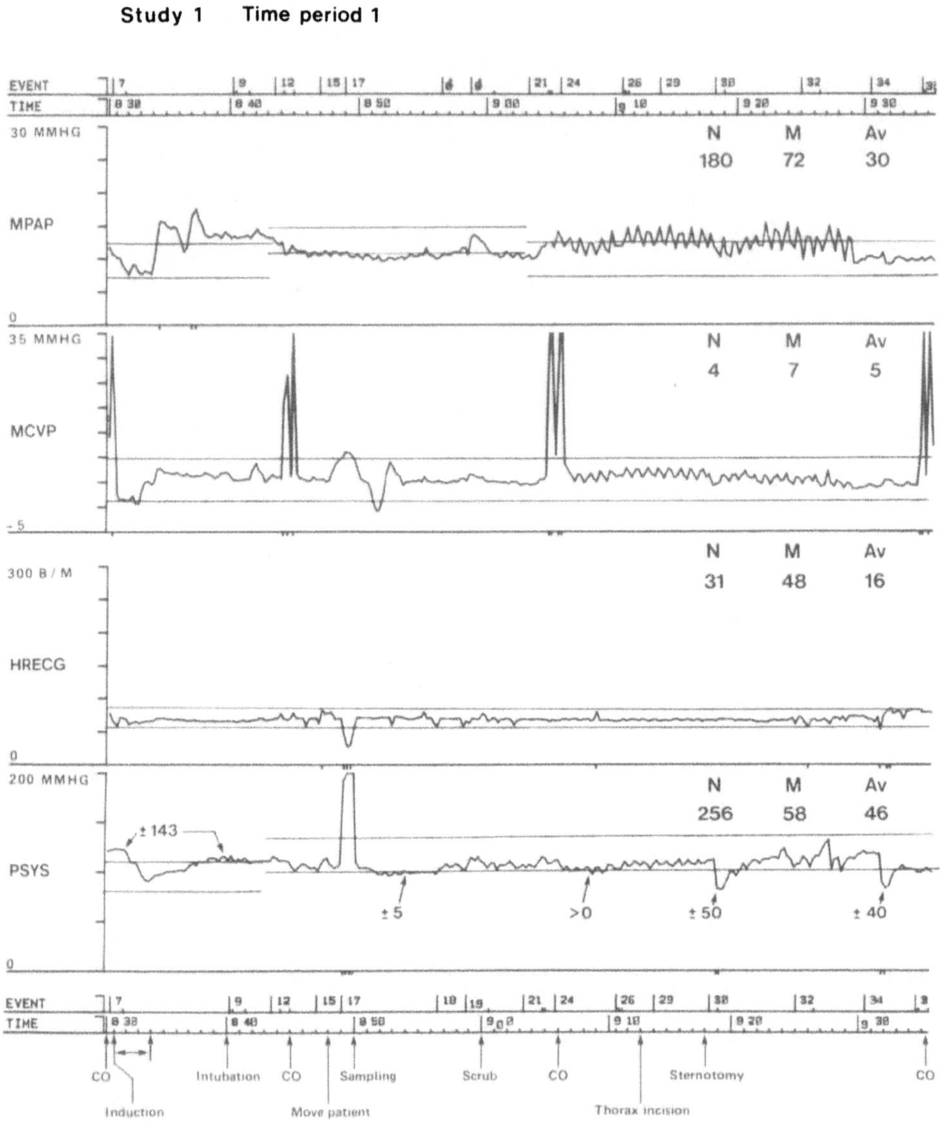

Fig. 5.11 Note:
- Relatively high N value for PSYS due to a number of minor transgressions of the zone (compositing surfaces marked with arrows).
- Rise in MPAP at induction.
- Considerable fluctuations in MCVP around 8h50, cause unknown.
- Oscillating signal behavior in the blood pressures starting at 9h06, cause unknown.

Study 1 Time period 2

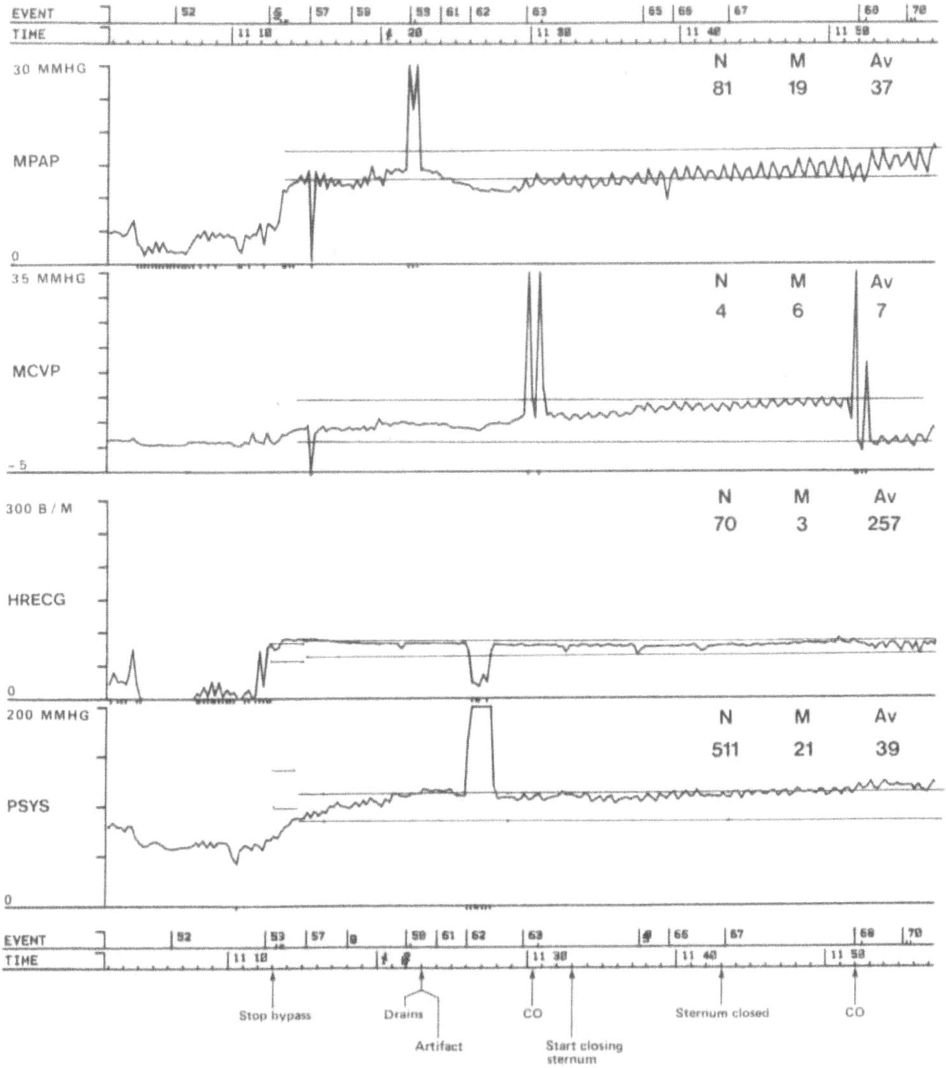

Fig. 5.12 Note:

- High N value for PSYS due to many minor transgressions of the zone.
- High AV value for HR; because of the long time constants used for computation of $\bar{x}_k$ and d_k these values lag far behind the actual signal behavior at the point where bypass is suddenly stopped.
- Same oscillatory phenomena.

Study 2 Time period 1

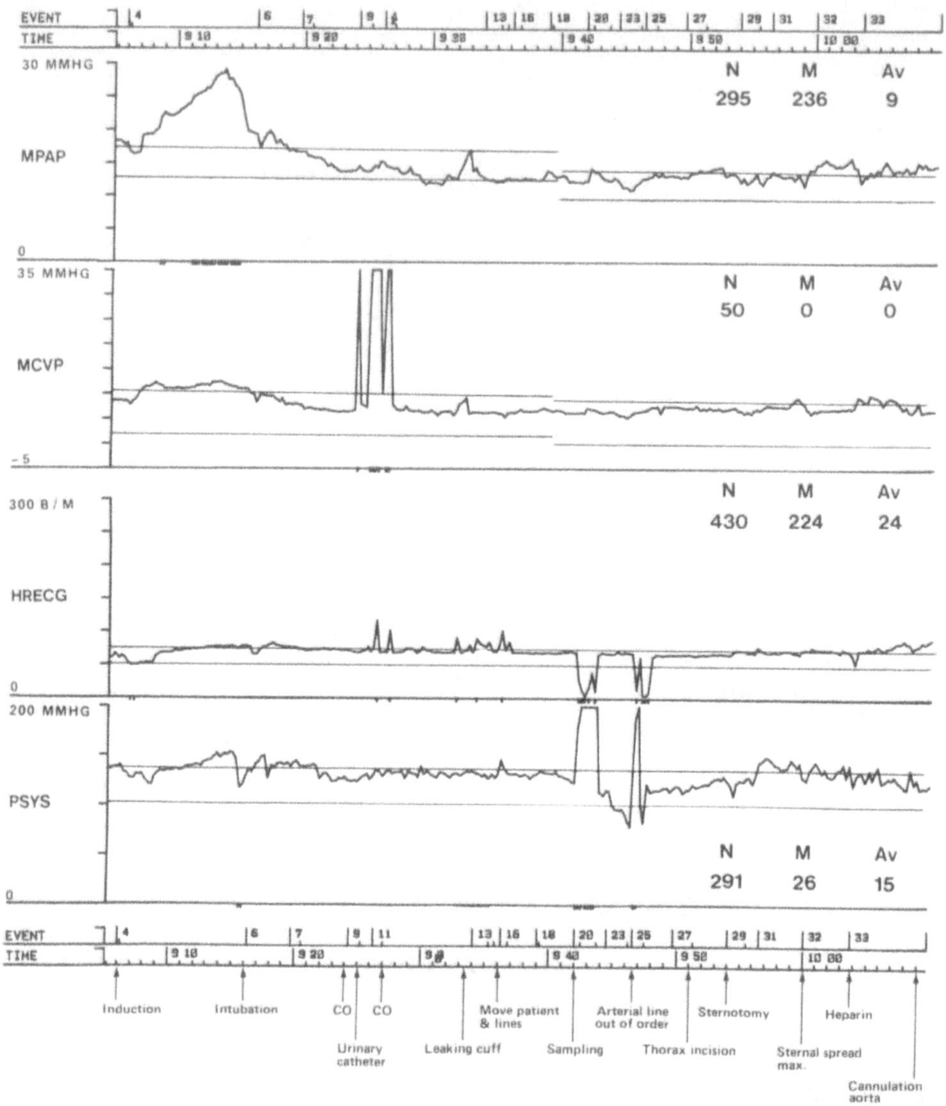

Fig. 5.13 Note:
- High N,M,AV values for HR; HR is low resulting in narrow bands around norm and mean. This results in a large surface area which is created by the many minor fluctuations in an otherwise stable signal.
- High N,M values for MPAP mainly caused by the rise in MPAP at induction.

Study 2 Time period 2

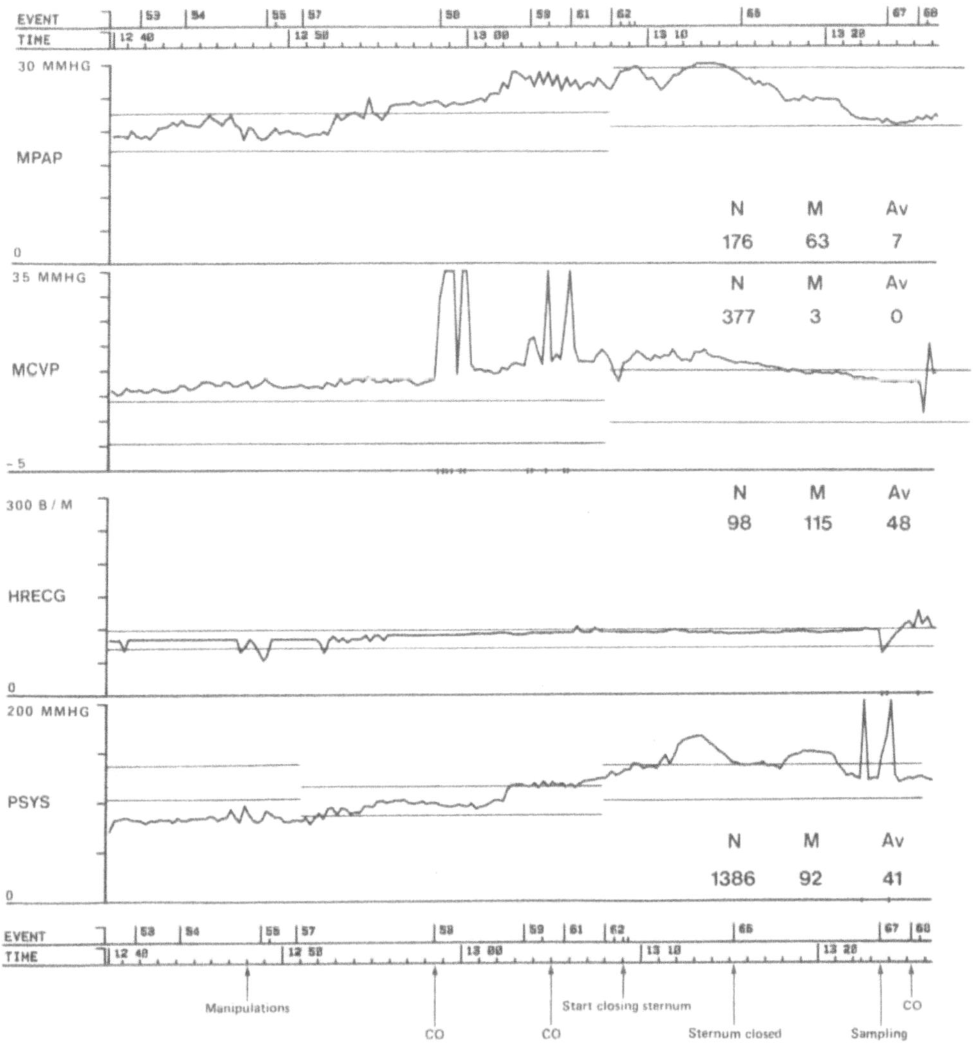

Fig. 5.14 Note:

- Consistent trend in PSYS resulting in a high N value while the M value is much smaller because it was computed over the three different norm intervals.
- High (clinically unacceptable) absolute level of MCVP resulting in high N value.
- Enormous rise in MPAP level in comparison with first time period (T1).

Study 14 Time period 1

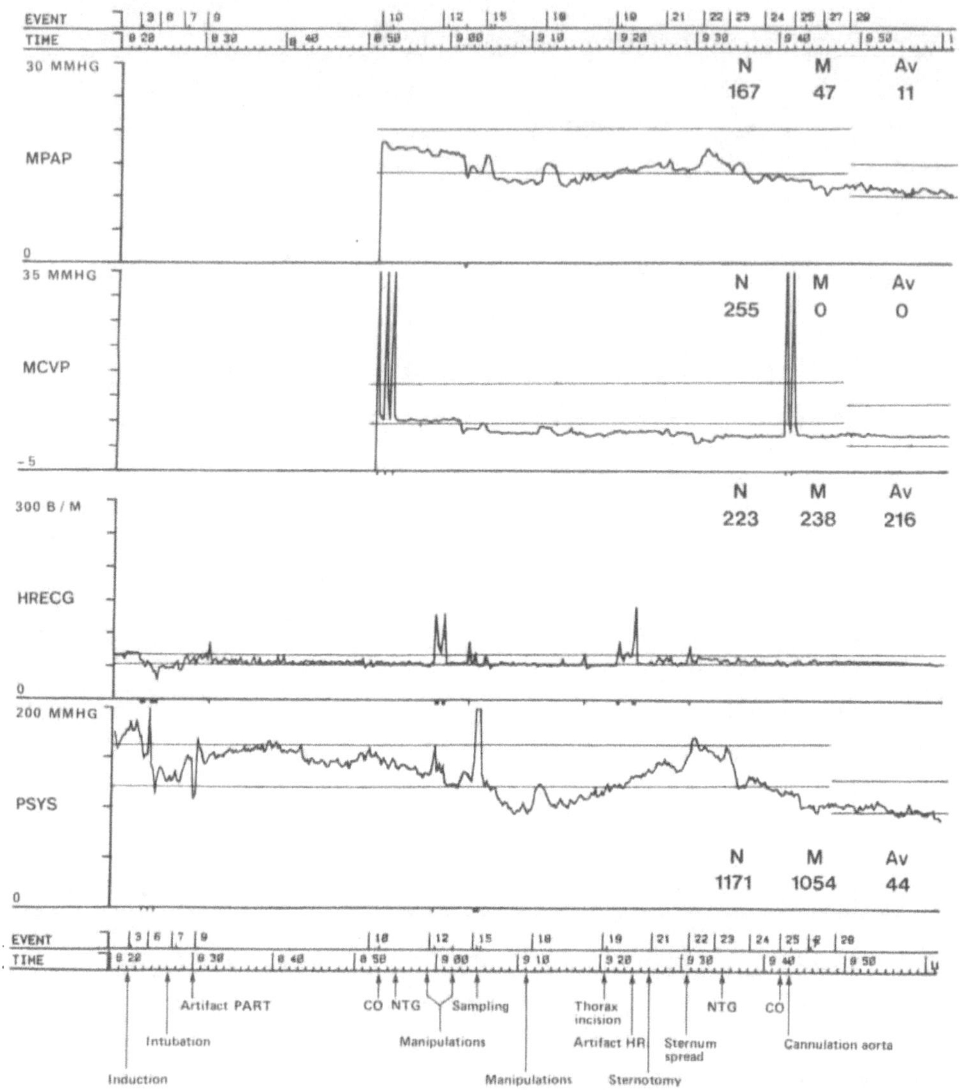

Fig. 5.15 Note:

- Unstable PSYS resulting in high N and M level apparently $\bar{x}_k$ could trace the trends and thus AV is not high.
- Large N value for MCVP versus zero M level caused by wrong setting of norm value.

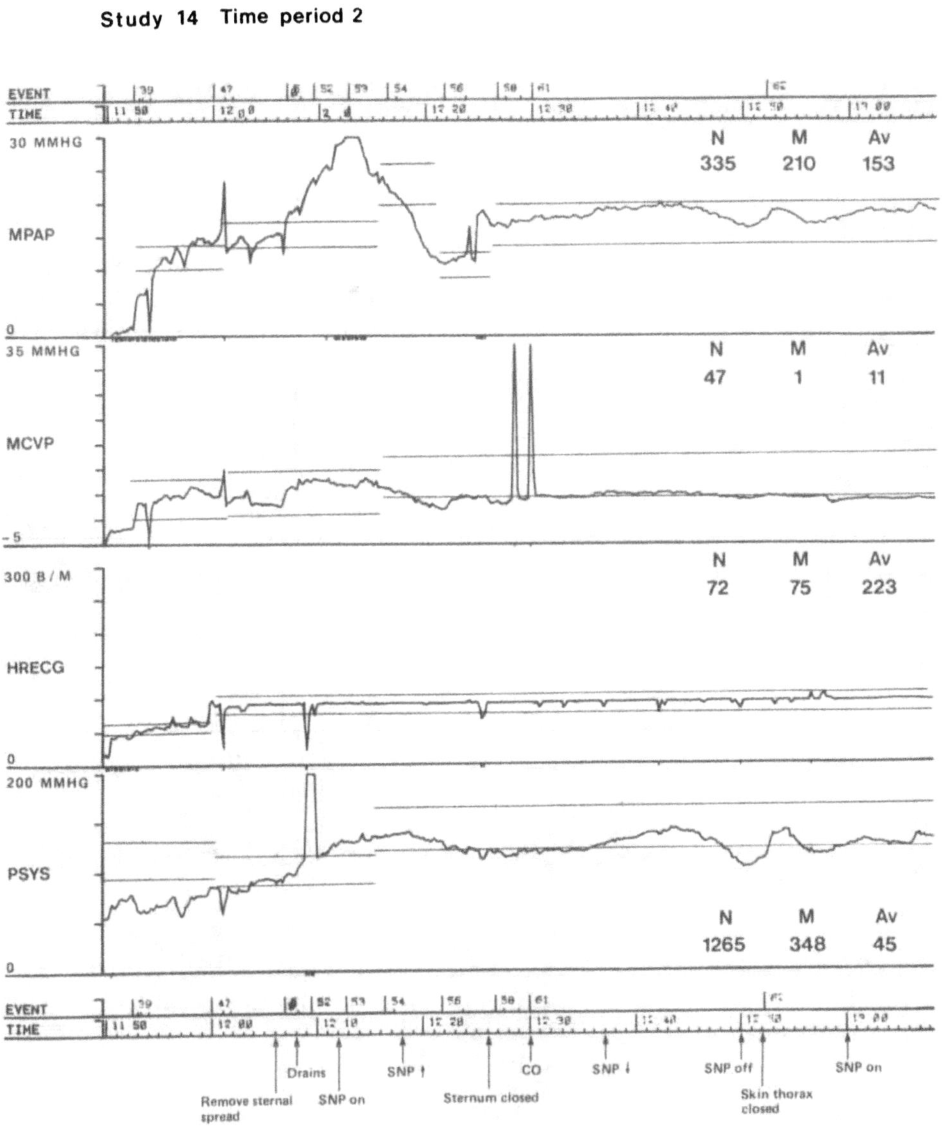

Fig. 5.16 Note:
- Frequent rescaling of MPAP and still high N, M and AV levels; cause of signal behavior around 12h15 unknown.

Study 16 Time period 1

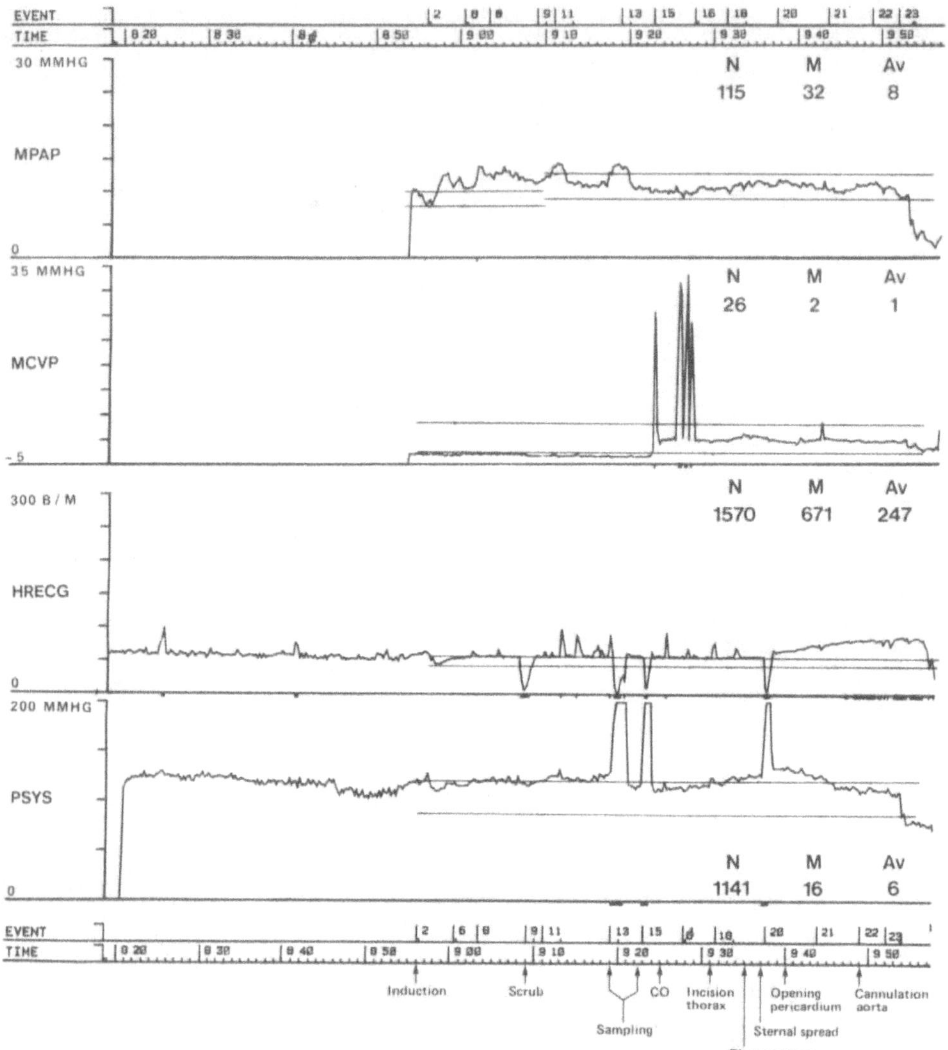

Fig. 5.17 Note:

- High N versus low M value for PSYS.
- High N,M,AV values for HR caused amongst other things by trend starting around 9h38.
- Unstable HR in relation to second time period.

Study 16 Time period 2

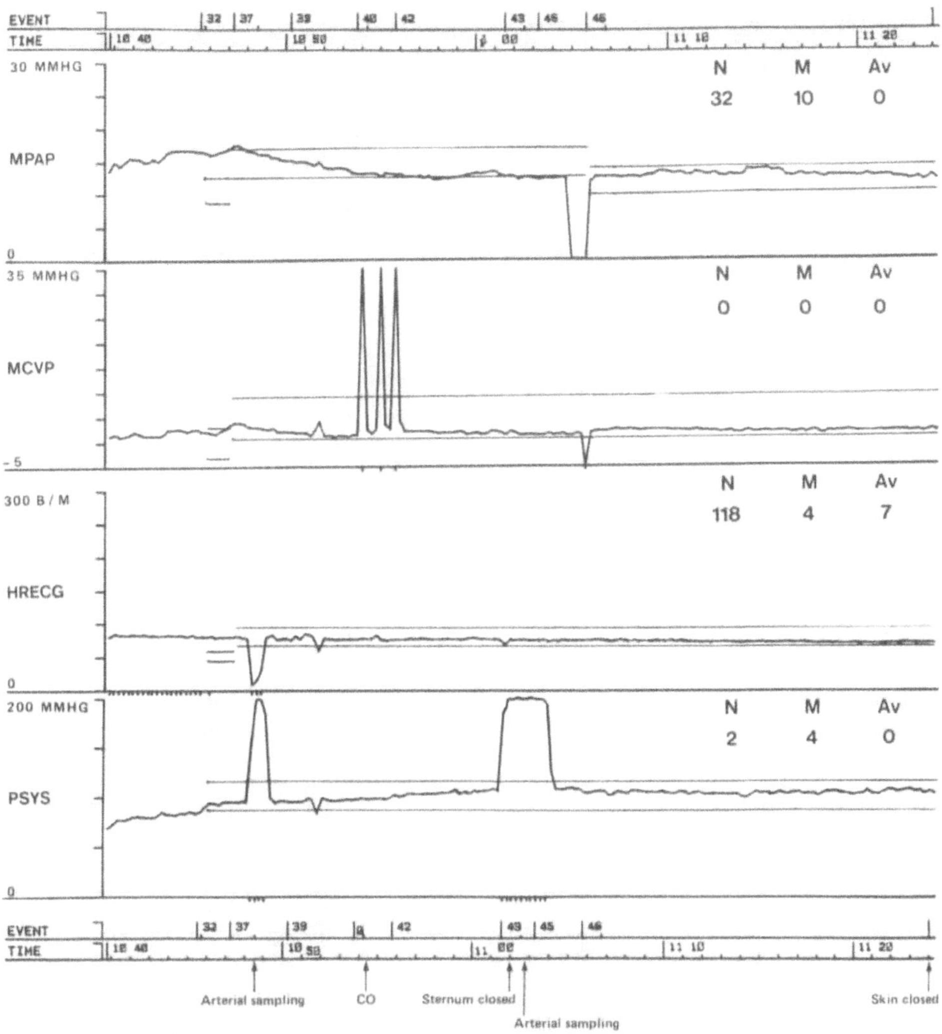

Fig. 5.18 Note:
- Remarkably stable signals.

Study 20 Time period 1

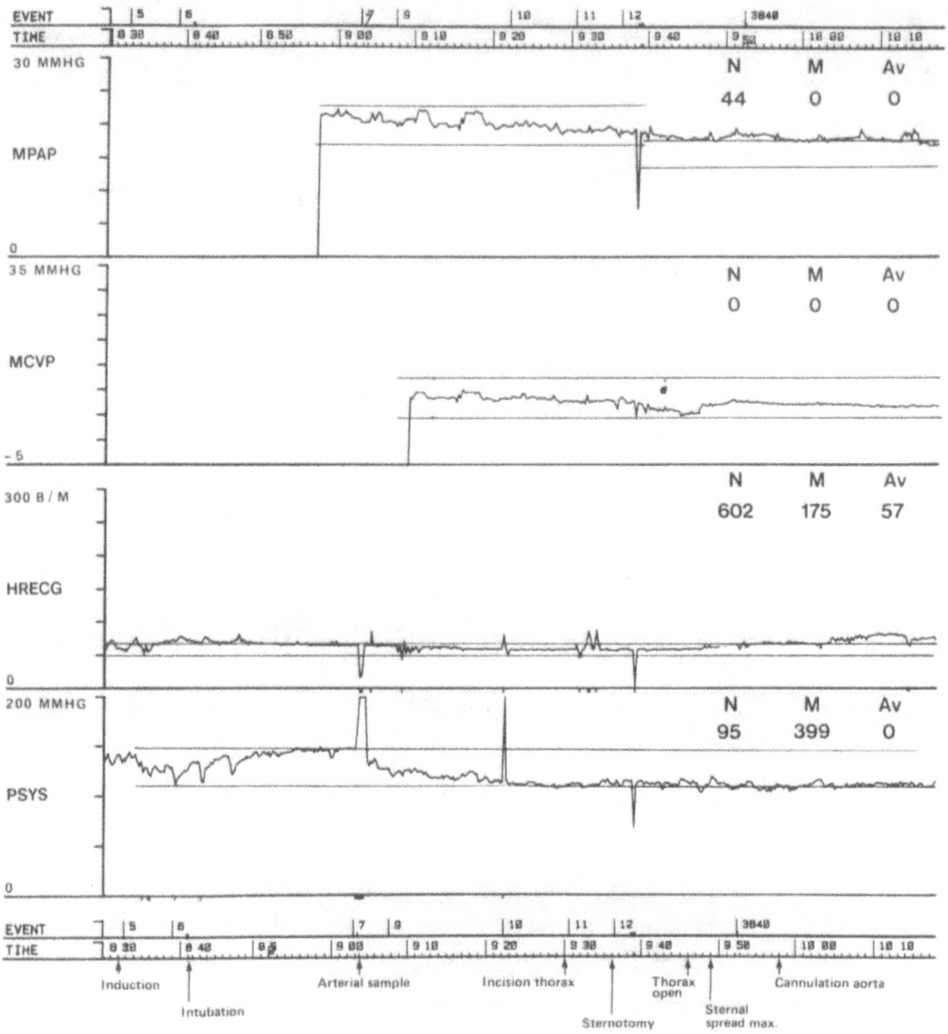

Fig. 5.19 Note:

- M> >N for PSYS because of trends in PSYS, sometimes such a surface in M is also small because the norm value was rescaled. Rescaling implies at the same time the start of a new interval over which M is computed. In this sample no rescaling was done.

true, but the small sample size is a factor of more importance. With a small sample size it is difficult to detect small differences between the subpopulations. When no difference is detected this does not necessarily mean that no difference is present. There is a chance β which increases with decreasing sample size that a certain difference stays undetected (Freiman et al. 1978). For normal distributions this chance can be computed and at an α of 0.05 and a sample size of 30 the chance that a shift of 10% is missed is about 80%. For the nonparametric tests which had to be applied in this study this chance β is still greater.

Apart from the sample size, a factor which probably obscures the possible shifts in controllability even more, is the enormous variability in the controllability values. For instance, over the thirty patients the error of control in the PSYS ranges from 100 to 2500. An attempt was made to detect factors which may cause the variability. From scanning the relevant patient data, e.g. age, sex, premedication, and preoperative blood pressures, it followed that the blood pressure upon arrival in the operating room might be a factor of influence. Therefore a Wilcoxon/Mann-Whitney test was applied to detect whether a high blood pressure (PSYS ≥ 160mmHg and/or PDIA ≥ 95mmHg), determined as the mean over five minutes before induction, has a significant ($p < 0.05$) influence on the controllability of the arterial pressures. Of these tests 21% were significant, with 17% concerning the controllability in the first time period. Thus the controllability is, among other things, strongly related to the blood pressure before induction. From this fact we can derive the suggestion that in a later study, variability might be diminished by trying to regulate these patients with a high blood pressure better by means of a stronger premedication.

If the assumption from which we departed, that a lower error of control might be related to improved patient care is true, this adjustment of premedication should also be in the interest of the patients (Schneider et al. 1979).

However, this assumption can be made the subject of extensive discussions. Of course most major or long-lasting fluctuations are undesirable. But it is also undesirable that the reflexes of a patient should be suppressed more than required. For each patient a threshold value exists. It is the art of anesthesia to balance around this threshold (see Section 2.2). With this and comparable studies, perhaps support can be given in the peroperative determination of this optimal threshold for each patient.

5.4 Summary

With the studies described in this chapter we tried to determine objectively the degree of influence of DADS on the course of anesthesia. Two tests were developed and applied: the first regarded the disturbance detection algorithm of DADS and the second measured the "controllability" of anesthesia.

In the first test it was investigated whether the new warning method of DADS indeed warns for signal changes which are clinically significant. This was done by determining the relevance of the warnings after observation of the related actions of the medical staff. The method of investigation worked satisfactorily. It led to the conclusion that between 7% and 12% of the warnings are useful. If a number of artifacts is suppressed this number can increase to between 8% and 15%. Although these useful warnings are very important for the detection of critical incidents, they are still obscured by a considerable number of useless warnings. Moreover, there are about 10 useful warnings per procedure which are not detected by the algorithm. Several measures are planned to improve the contribution of useful warnings, such as the automated system input of medical interventions, the use of signal correlations, and further artifact suppression. Although the warning algorithm needs further improvement, the method which was followed to obtain the significance of the warnings is a useful approach to objectively charting anesthesia management.

The second test regarded the so-called controllability of anesthesia. The degree to which the deviation of signals with respect to their normal band is influenced by DADS as opposed to the conventional monitoring equipment was investigated. For the small population which was studied no significant influence of DADS could be shown.

The error of control was not significantly lowered but certainly not heightened either; there were some minor tendencies which pointed in favor of DADS.

The cases with a lower error of control were found mostly in the period after bypass. This seems in the first instance to be caused by a more stable state of the patient.

Although the controllability measure was not sufficiently sensitive to show an influence of DADS, it did show some difference in controllability between the three anesthesiologists who participated in the study. Also, with this second performance test, interesting relationships between interventions and signal behavior can be detected. The most striking signal pattern was the strong (uncontrollable) rise in mean pulmonary arterial pressure at induction.

6 Evaluation: Redesign Considerations

6.1 Introduction

In this chapter we will deal with Step 3 and Step 5 of the evaluation method as composed in Chapter 4. These steps concern the so-called redesign or improvement phase. For this phase the designers needed information covering all minor and major missions and aspects of DADS, ranging from the reliability of the bits of the display memories to the value of the design philosophy of the bar display. In order to obtain a complete picture of all the suggestions, remarks and ideas regarding either the properties of DADS or new requirements for DADS, a checklist was composed consisting of the minor and major items of interest. As an example, item 14 of the checklist, which concerns the graphical display, is given in Table 6.1.

The use of such a checklist guarantees that attention is given to all ideas which arise and that the risk of paying too much attention to a specific idea just because it is frequently mentioned by one person can be obviated. The checklist concerns both technical, ergonomical and utility aspects; in this chapter the ergonomic aspects will be dealt with. Until now, the research which has been done into operating room ergonomics concerns aspects such as illumination and colors with respect to surgical requirements (Putsep 1979) or the influence of climatic conditions on the performance of the medical staff (Graafmans 1986). However, our present interest concerns the work situation of the anesthesiologist and, more specifically, the ergonomic requirements which apply when color monitors are included in the monitoring equipment. As yet not much of this knowledge has been systematically applied to the work situation of the anesthesiologist in the OR.

Three subjects of major importance will be discussed:

- man-machine interaction (Section 6.2)
- data presentation (Section 6.3)
- equipment layout (the integrated workstation) (Section 6.4).

6.2 Ergonomics: Man-Machine Interaction

This section deals with the results of the evaluation with respect to the man-machine interaction between the user and DADS; this topic required extra attention according to Döring (1976a) (Section 4.3). The interaction protocol of DADS was described in Section 3.5, it includes both commands to operate the system, e.g. to

Table 6.1 Checklist of evaluation items for the graphical display

14. The graphical display:
- 14.1 Layout (q,i)*
  - 14.1.1 More and/or other possibilities required
    - 14.1.1.1 More grids
    - 14.1.1.2 Variables against each other
  - 14.1.2 Colors (n,q,i)
    - 14.1.2.1 Rod graph
    - 14.1.2.2 Line graph
    - 14.1.2.3 Axes
    - 14.1.2.4 Names
  - 14.1.3 Location of scale values (q,i)
  - 14.1.4 Division of the axes
  - 14.1.5 Present value presentation
  - 14.1.6 Principle of the possibility to select different scale values for the various variables
- 14.2 Status identification
- 14.3 Time axis (q,i,n)
  - 14.3.1 Presentation
  - 14.3.2 Lengths
  - 14.3.3 Other possibilities **
- 14.4 Use
  - 14.4.1 Access frequency
  - 14.4.2 Presentation time
    - 14.4.2.1 Automatic change-over to other displays required (q,i)?
  - 14.4.3 Used graph compositions
- 14.5 Readability (i,q,n)
  - 14.5.1 From what distance
  - 14.5.2 Character size
  - 14.5.3 Symbol density
- 14.6 Update frequency (i,q)

* The characters in brackets give an indication as to which techniques (in order of importance) are the most suitable for obtaining the information on the subject (Section 4.3): i stands for interview, q for questionnaire, n for nonobtrusive methods, s for self-observation, o for observation. For example the requirements on legibility can be found unobtrusively by applying the ergonomic literature to the properties of the displayed information. However, by interviewing the users or submitting questionnaires, valuable information can also be obtained.

** DADS presents graphs on a small number of time scales with the end point always at the present value. Another possibility would be to give a free choice in both begin and end times of the graphs.

change the presented information, and free or structured comments with information about the surgical procedure. The device used for interaction is a keyboard equipped with an additional set of function keys. In Section 3.8 some of the different types of comments were listed. They concern events, drug administration, blood gas values and electrolytes, fluid balance information, etc. Schneider (1982) determined that a complete anesthetic record requires at least forty of these time-independent entries for each procedure, with an additional eight per hour duration of the procedure. It is likely that, with the progress in automation of clinical laboratories, the values which are initially determined outside the OR will become available for automated reading by DADS. Others will certainly follow when more uniformity in measuring equipment is realized. However, at the moment all these values have to be entered by means of the keyboard. To reduce the workload required for entry of these data in DADS, a special extension to the interaction protocol has been designed for improving the efficiency of their input and presentation (Section 3.8). This extension requires the keyboard to be expanded with an additional 20 keys to a total of approximately 50 function keys. Though Galer and Yap (1980) cite a study where it was demonstrated that subjects may operate successfully when 137 keys are used, Oborne (1985, p91) mentions some studies where other input devices were shown to be more efficient for a simple task such as the selecting of an item from a screen.

During the use of DADS in the operating room the operators also detected some drawbacks in the interaction by means of the keyboard. One of these concerned the scaling of the bar display. In Fig. 6.1 a time line of a surgical procedure is given. During this period, the operator tried to maintain an optimal setting of the bar display. This means that norm value and alarm values were adapted timely to a new (acceptable) state of patient signals. In this case the bar display had to be rescaled 12 times.

In the studies described in Section 5.3, where rescaling was allowed only sparingly, the average rescaling rate was 4 over the two time slices, excluding the bypass phase. Every rescale action requires about 15 keystrokes. In both situations time and attention required for these key strokes were considered to be too much. It has been suggested that manipulation of the limits on the screen with the finger tip could be a solution. For this a "touch screen" would be required.

The remarks regarding keyboard drawbacks as stated above, combined with the possibilities which may be offered by alternative devices, led us to perform a study in which the total man-machine interaction was reviewed.

The following steps were taken:

- After inclusion of possible additional commands an inventory was made of the *interaction facilities* (6.2.1);
- The possible *interaction protocols* were studied (software) (6.2.2);
- The existing *input devices* were studied (hardware) (6.2.3);

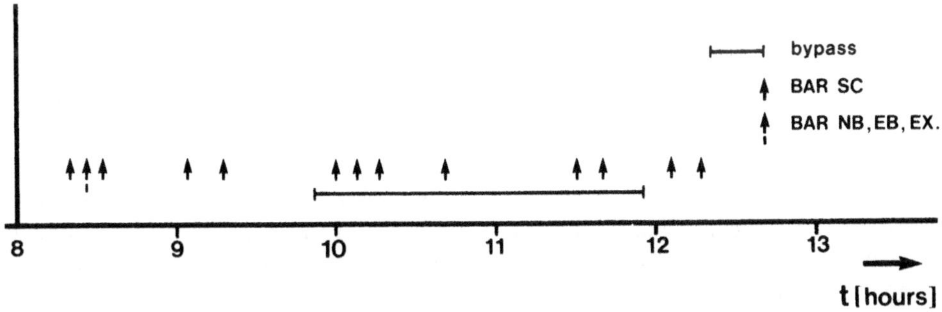

Fig. 6.1 During an anesthetic procedure lasting 5 hours, the operator rescaled the bar display as often as required for an optimal presentation of the signals. Twelve rescale operations were performed.

- Possible combinations of input device and interaction protocol were made resulting in *proposals for improved interaction* (6.2.4).

In the sections below these steps will be discussed as far as relevant for DADS.

6.2.1 The Interaction Facilities

As mentioned above, the list of requirements for DADS was checked. This provided us with a number of minor points for improvement.

Because these improvements require commands in addition to the set which was given in Section 3.5, some of these will be mentioned below :

- A type of display will be added to the facilities of DADS in which two variables can be plotted against each other (GRAPH VARIABLE), e.g. left atrial pressure against the administered fluids. A command will be required to call for this new display format.
- For each user it will be possible to define and save several display versions; so different displays can be saved for different procedures or patients, etc. This will require on-line save and call functions.
- In the GRAPH SINGLE and DOUBLE display, an event bar and a cursor line will be introduced.
  The event bar enables exact readout of the relationship between interventions and signal behavior.
  The cursor line can be positioned at a place in the plot where readout of time and signal values is desired; this entails that a means to move the cursor line must be available.
- It must be possible to choose freely the beginning and end of the interval over which a GRAPH has to be plotted. Although this will require additional entry of these times, no extra provisions have to be made.
- Some commands are added to enhance the consistency between the bar and graph commands.
  In Fig. 6.2 the interaction facilities, including the supplementary commands, are listed.

Both the information as presented by DADS (machine output -> human input) and the input of control and medical data (human output-> machine input) are given, and the commands are subdivided into categories. Apart from the supplementary commands some new categories were also included:

- Within the scope of the integrated workstation it is our opinion that, at a later stage, the category "Instrument Control" should be expanded, for instance with commands to adjust the settings on a ventilator. If this is realized it is probable that an additional category will be necessary which presents "Control Related Data" to the user.
- The category "Data Management" is also new. It comprises instructions for obtaining off-line access to the stored data, e.g. those necessary for composing a list for information transfer to the ICU.

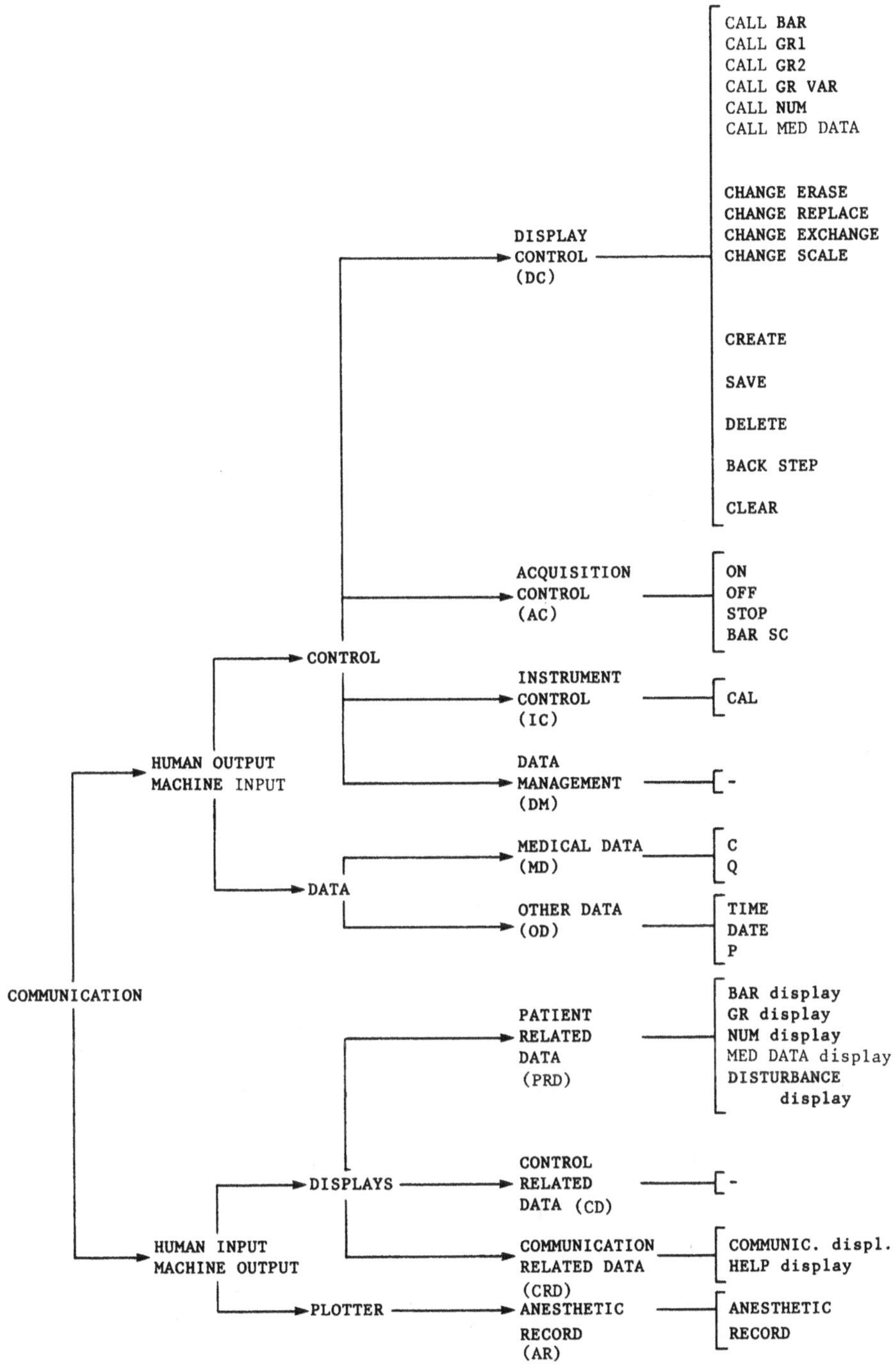

Fig. 6.2 The interaction facilities encompass in fact both the human output-> machine input, such as control commands and data entry, and the machine output-> human input that is, the information presentation. Improvements for the latter will be given in Section 6.3.

- The category "Other Data" contains commands to call for time and date and for entering "private comments" which will not be listed in a standard report. These commands already have been implemented. Additionally, in this category, extensions are planned which will enable the user to perform simple arithmetic such as converting a drug concentration from mg/kg/min to ml/hour as must be set on the pump.

The elements of such a command set partially determine the requirements to be met by the input devices and the interaction protocol. For instance free comments cannot be entered by means of function keys or with a protocol in which only a choice can be made from items on a list (menus). Because of its variety the category "Medical Data" in particular makes high demands upon the choice of input device(s) and interaction protocol.

6.2.2 *The Interaction Protocol*

The current interaction with DADS is basically userdriven (Kasuga 1982): the user has to enter a command and the system (re)acts accordingly. The overall command structure is a tree with branches and nodes. Every command is a composition of a main command, a subcommand and a set of arguments (Section 3.5). When a user enters an incomplete or faulty command, the protocol switches to the "system driven" mode in which the user is prompted by an elucidating question to enter the next segment of the command. The available command options in every node of the command tree can be displayed by means of the HELP facility (menu presentation). In the planned extension for entry of the medical data some additional interaction facilities had to be applied to ensure efficiency. For the entry of events and drugs the user can choose from menus; the realized menu software is such that the most likely entry from the list gets the highest priority in the menu and is presented first. Next, when for instance a drug has been chosen from the drug menu, a kind of form-filling protocol is started which enables the user to enter the numerical value of the dose in a preformatted line.

This interaction protocol, though rather diverse in its components, is very logical. Smooth and efficient data and command entry is realized by automatic switching from one protocol principle to another. This was confirmed during the clinical evaluation of DADS. Apart from the lack of a line editor, no major problems were encountered with the protocol and user satisfaction was sufficient. Therefore it was decided not to revise the interaction protocol but to restrict ourselves to improvements and adjustments required by the choice of new input devices.

6.2.3 *Input Devices*

Although an interaction protocol has to be adapted to the hardware input device(s), minor and sometimes major adjustments are possible and, depending on the flexibility of the software, easy to implement. However, once a hardware device has been selected, the choice is more or less final and cannot easily be changed. Perhaps this is one of the reasons that in the ergonomic literature much attention is paid to hardware. Several authors spend extensive discussions on the (dis)advantages of the various input devices (Oborne 1985, Murray 1981).

Therefore, we shall cover the existing hardware devices only briefly with respect to their suitability for the monitoring environment and for DADS in particular. General remarks regarding the functionality of the devices are cited from Oborne (1985) and Murray (1981).

Several input devices are currently available or under development:

1. Touch sensitive devices
2. Pointing devices
3. Positioning devices
4. Keyboard devices
5. Reading devices
6. Speech recognizing devices

When discussing the suitability of input devices for DADS we must keep the following considerations in mind.

In the current prototype of DADS, information presentation takes place on color monitors. Because of the limited space available in the operating room, input devices should require as little additional space as possible.

It became clear from Fig. 6.2 and the accompanying discussion that globally two kinds of commands are required for interaction with DADS: simple, uniform commands for operating the system, consisting of a main command, a sub command and a set of arguments, and medical data with a format strongly depending on the character of these data. In correspondence with the current implementation using a keyboard for interaction, we maintained the starting point that to enhance user-friendly interaction, new device(s) should enable permanent presentation of the first two levels of the commands. Furthermore, until the level of automation reaches a suitable level of advancement, it will be necessary to invest in special devices which facilitate medical data entry.

ad 1: Touch-Sensitive Devices: These include all the devices where input takes place by pointing at preprogrammed data-items, with or without an aid. The most important examples are, the touch-screen and the graphics tablet.

Trispel and Rau (1982) developed a so-called Anesthesia Information System (AIS). In the design of this system the emphasis was put on a new method of man-machine interaction in the operating room by means of a touch screen. In the interaction several favorable properties of the touch screen are employed.

+ On a single screen the course of automatically sampled data is presented in graphs alongside space reserved for entry of standard medical data. The entry of medical data is performed by choosing from menus. Usually two menus, one level apart, are presented on one screen. One "key" is always reserved for going back to the main menu.
+ Different colors are applied for the presentation of the (sub)commands/data on a certain level; one color is used to show the items which are activated.

From the activated items, one can be selected for entry in accordance with the command structure. The entry of a specific item is then acknowledged with another color, and a third color is used to indicate the items which cannot be entered at that node in the command structure.

+ On their touch screen "manipulation techniques" are also applied. "Virtual control elements" such as a dial or a slide can be programmed to appear on the screen. The simulated dial or pointer can be adjusted by sliding with the fingertip over the screen. Thus the highest input resolution possible for the screen is reached because each touch-sensitive location can be activated and has its own numerical value.

It occurs quite frequently that the time at which a certain intervention is entered into the system does not correspond with the time of the intervention itself. Therefore it is important to provide the user with an easy means of entering this time afterwards. In the AIS this is realized by enabling the user to place the cursor line in the signal graph at the time corresponding with a medical intervention. In this way exact entry of the time is possible.

The main limitation of such a touch screen is that the entry of free alphanumerical text is not possible. Furthermore it is considered to be a tedious job to enter series of data. Special attention is required when positioning a touch screen in the work environment; the user must have a view perpendicular to the screen since otherwise the relation between the presented data item and the touch sensitive spot may be lost (parallax).

The other important pointing device is the graphics tablet. Newbower et al. (1981a) incorporated the graphics tablet in a prototype system for data entry in computer-assisted record-keeping. In this system data entry takes place by entering the data on a modified, but fairly standard, anesthesia record placed on the surface of the tablet, thus combining data entry and conventional record keeping. The recognition of characters by the tablet is facilitated by dividing the tablet into different active areas: one area for plotting the course of 9 "vital signs" by means of 9 different symbols which are recognized by the tablet so that the course of the signals can be stored automatically, and another area reserved for drug and fluid administration. The name of a drug is entered by touching the name in a list on the record. The entry of doses is accomplished by writing the appropriate value numerically in line with the previously entered drug name and with the correct time of administration. The remaining information is entered in yet another area.

In this example all data are entered manually. It is also possible to plot automatically sampled data on a record and enter the remaining data manually on the same record. Such a device for semi-automated record keeping was designed by Gravenstein and Paulus (1986) and is commercially available.

Since, for DADS, flexible data presentation by means of color monitors is the starting point, the use of a graphics tablet would have the disadvantage that the setup is more extensive; besides, it does not seem logical to enter commands to control the presentation on the monitors via a separately positioned graphics tablet. For procedures where flexible data presentation is not required, where manual data entry is favored for reasons of vigilance, or where automated data sampling is not available, the graphics tablet seems a very suitable device. With progressively improving techniques for the recognition of handwriting, its use will become less restricted to symbols; this will eventually make its application more common.

ad 2: Pointing Devices: A device which is comparable to the mouse, in that it can be used to select items on a screen, and to the touch screen in that coordinates of the selected item are recorded, is the lightpen. It is a pencil-shaped device which is mainly suitable for the tracking of lines in order to enter their coordinates into a computer. Its application is, among other things, found in systems for computer-aided design, where the attention of the operator has to be directed only to the screen. Its application is not suitable for DADS.

ad 3: Positioning Devices: Apart from the well-known cursor control keys implemented on almost every keyboard, there are other devices which can be used to position a cursor on a data item which is to be entered, erased or replaced, or which has to be indicated for other reasons, e.g. because knowledge on that specific subject is required. The most important examples are the joystick and the "mouse".

The mouse is the newest positioning device. It has the shape of a pack of cigarettes, is attached to the computer and can be moved with a very high precision in every direction over a flat surface. The cursor moves correspondingly on the screen.

A joystick requires much less space but does not allow the same precision: a small movement with the joystick may result in a large movement of the cursor.

Whatever device may be chosen as the most appropriate, the positioning of a cursor takes more time than a single key entry and it is an additional control task which directs attention away from the patient. Therefore, its application is only useful when it can replace the regular entry of several keystrokes, as in the system described by Trispel and Rau (1982) where the entry of time is not needed.

ad 4: Keyboard Devices: These include all devices where entry takes place by means of keys, varying from the commonly used alphanumerical keyboard to function keyboards and softkeys.

By means of the alphanumerical keyboard all data can be entered and all interaction protocols are possible. However, for entry of only one item, e.g. the name of a drug, quite a few key strokes may be required, with the possibility that errors occur, resulting in low efficiency.

A function keyboard consists of keys with a fixed meaning, for entry of an item which otherwise would require a few keyboard entries. Function keyboards are easy and fast to operate and do not need any special skill. Typing errors cannot occur and thus the reproduction of entries on the screen is not necessary, although a provision for acknowledging an operation is advisable.

However, function keyboards are static hardware devices with the only flexibility that other functions can be assigned to the keys. Mainly because of the number of different medical data which must be entered, the control of a monitoring system such as DADS would at the moment require too many function keys. Therefore, function keys are currently not suitable to be the only means for command entry.

Pads with softkeys are in fact function keyboards with a limited set of keys, the meaning of which can be changed depending on the node in the command structure. The momentary meaning of the key is presented on a display adjacent to the keys. Softkeys are easy and fast to operate, and flexible; the number of keys can be limited even in elaborate applications. However, some space on the display is required to present the meaning of the keys. For every step in a command, a selection is possible from only a limited set of data items. The corresponding interaction protocol will thus be mostly menu-based; free commands and comments are not possible.

ad 5: Reading Devices: Some preoperatively obtained data such as demographic data and data from the medical history of the patients are essential for a computerized monitoring system in the operating room to enable complete record generation and 'intelligent' alarms.

Apart from typing and the possibilities as provided by automation (communication lines, floppy disks) these data can be stored on special information carriers such as bar codes and magnetic cards. By means of the corresponding reading device the information can be simply retrieved and stored by the monitoring system. This method of data entry may also be suitable for peroperative data: Trispel et al. (1981) performed a test to compare the speed of data entry concerning blood infusions by means of the touch-screen-based protocol of their AIS and a bar code reader. With the latter technique, the time for entries regarding blood infusions was reduced to 30% of the original time.

A bar code reader was extensively applied in the automated patient-monitoring system as described by Block et al. (1985). In the "DAME" system all data which could not be collected automatically were allotted a bar code and were entered by means of a bar code reader. The data included commands to change the display, standard comments, and administered drugs. This extensive application of the bar code scanner was unsuccessful: it was too much of a problem to select the appropriate bar code quickly. Also, bar codes were damaged because of their frequent use and the pressure exercised upon them during reading. Apart from this it followed that the bar code reader itself was rather vulnerable. Because of these disadvantages a bar code reader was not implemented in the second updated micro-DAME version. Still we think that the possibilities of bar code readers should be investigated further; for instance, bar codes could be applied to the labels on the drug syringes. In this way the entering of drug doses might be simplified and every code would still only be used once or twice.

ad 6: Speech Recognizing Devices: Sarnat et al. (1981) performed a preliminary evaluation of computerized speech recognition for anesthesia: a number of anesthesiologists were trained to use certain groups of words and short phrases. In sessions as yet outside the OR, the percentage of words recognized was determined. The overall recognition percentage was 95.9, which was judged as acceptable and therefore Sarnat (1983) is working on a subsequent, more powerful system. The advantage of speech entry is that it can be applied without suspension of the other (manual) tasks to be performed by the anesthesiologist: therefore in most cases, it will also be possible to enter the information at the exact time of occurrence of the intervention or event, and this is very advantageous for the accuracy of the anesthesia record. Although such devices are growing fast in importance, for the time being they are in too experimental a stage to be considered for implementation in DADS.

Conclusions: A number of currently available input devices was reviewed. With respect to their suitability for DADS we come to the following conclusions:

- Touch sensitive devices: The touch screen seems very suitable for implementation in DADS, but a solution must be found for the entry of free text. The graphics tablet requires too much additional space and is not sufficiently flexible.
- Pointing devices: These are not suitable for DADS.
- Positioning devices: Cursor positioning is necessary for some entries. The conventional cursor control keys need the least space.
- Keyboard devices: The function keys and softkey pads are both suitable for DADS but, again, a separate device would be required for the entry of free text.
- Reading devices: These seem suitable for transfer of data from outside the operating room into the system. In addition, such devices might also be used for a more objective method of entering drug administrations into the system (Section 8.2).
- Speech recognizing devices: These are as yet not sufficiently far developed. At a later stage they must certainly be subjected to further investigation.

6.2.4 Proposals for Improved Interaction

We concluded that the touch-screen, the keyboard devices and the cursor control keys seem to be the most suitable input media for DADS. We applied these devices in two proposals for improved interaction. The proposals will be illustrated by means of the control of some of the displays of DADS.

In the first proposal, DADS is equipped with a touch-screen and a row of function keys for each of the two color monitors. A third touch screen is applied for functioning as a virtual keyboard for entry of free text and the like.

In the second proposal the two monitors of DADS are equipped with a row of softkeys and a row of function keys. A keyboard is used for the remaining entries.

Proposal 1: When both monitors of DADS are equipped with a touch screen, this enables the application of manipulation techniques and complies with the interaction principle that commands regarding a specific screen must be entered at that screen (spatial compatibility, McCormick and Sanders 1983). The use of touch screens implies a menu-driven interaction protocol. This means that all the segments of a DADS command have to be entered step-by-step by activating the relevant item from the menu of the current level, which will result in a somewhat slower interaction because entry of a command in one line is no longer possible. Therefore it is important to prevent too many menu levels. Sisson (1983) recommended using not more than 2 or 3 levels. To realize this, a row of function keys is added to each touch-screen to present the main commands. In this way these keys are always available for switching to another display and the number of menu lev-

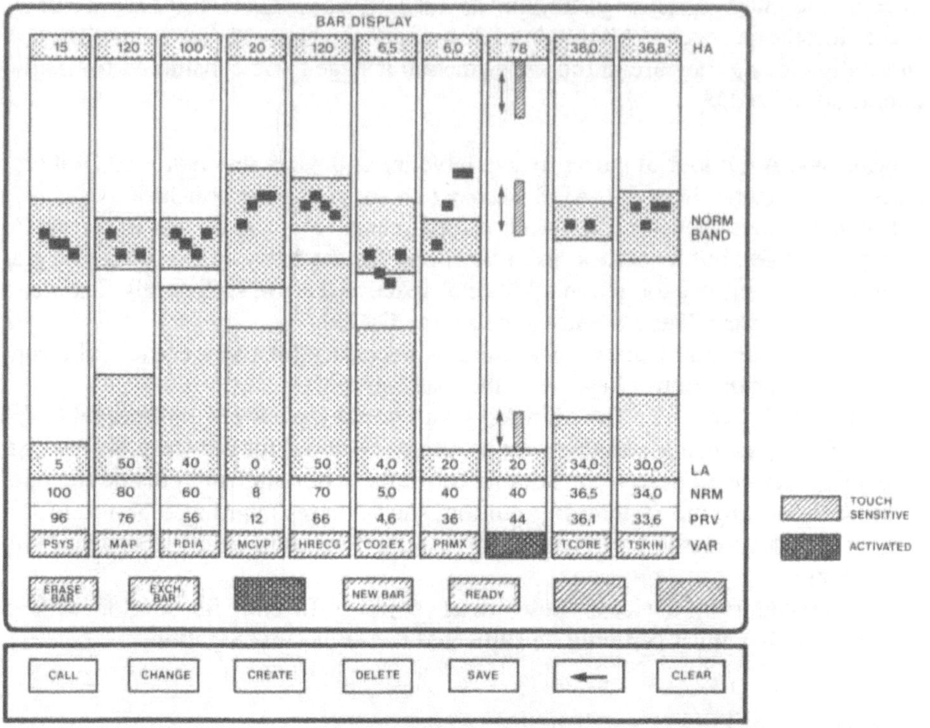

Fig. 6.3 A possible realization of the operation of the bar display by means of a touch-screen and a row of function keys. A function key is always available to CALL directly for a bar or graph display. Editing of the bar display takes place by means of two rows of virtual keys and manipulation techniques. In menu 1 the scale key was activated and the 8th bar was selected in menu 2 for rescaling. By manipulation, the relevant limits are adjusted directly on the screen.

els is decreased. In Fig. 6.3 a possible realization of the bar display and its operation by means of touch screen and function keys is presented.

Apart from the commands which directly concern the format of a display, some general commands for data acquisition and for entry of free comments are still needed. For these entries a common alphanumerical keyboard is almost indispensable. It has the advantage of low cost and tactile feedback. However, when a small, high-quality touch screen can be obtained, even this keyboard might be replaced.

Such a small touch screen can add considerably to surveyable interaction and display, and can be used interchangeably as a virtual alphanumerical keyboard to enable entry of free text, and as a virtual function keyboard for entering fixed medical data and for performing acquisition control operations (Fig. 6.4).

This results in a less interrupted data display on the lower monitor and, depending on the tasks which were allotted to the lower monitor, it may also reduce the number of menu levels for the lower monitor. Finally, it completes the separation of operation functions between the screens: the first and second monitors display selection and formatting, and the third screen shows medical data entry and acquisition control.

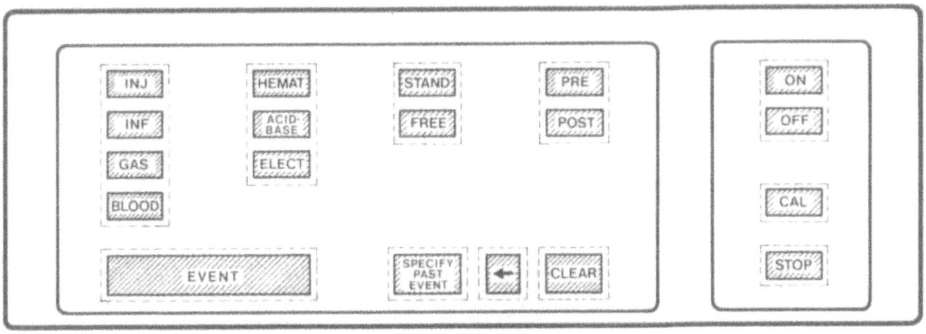

Fig. 6.4 In proposal 1, DADS is equipped with a third touch screen for entry of free text and other data such as medical data and acquisition control which do not explicitly belong to one of the screens.

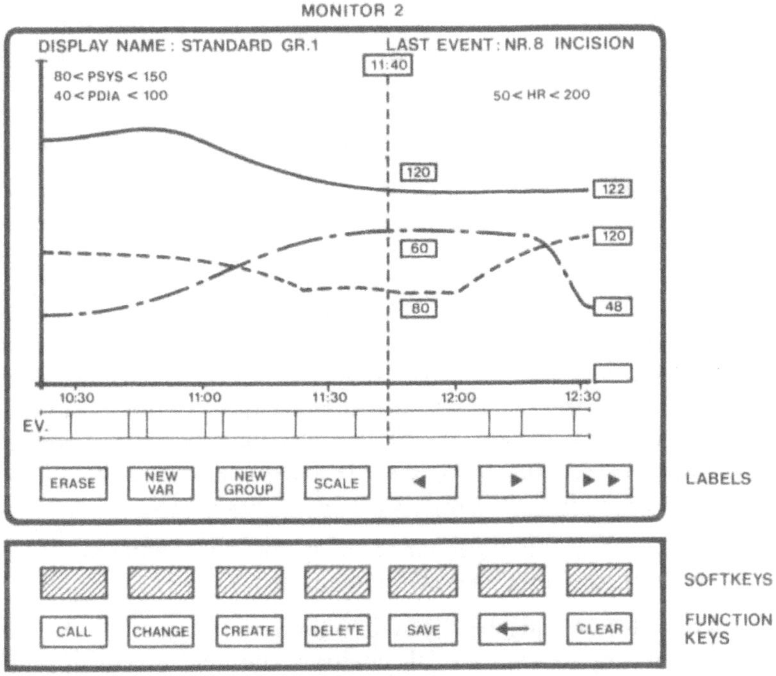

Fig. 6.5 The graphical display including new extensions such as the cursor line and a bar in which the events are presented. The display was retrieved by a call function and the labels of the softkeys have here the meaning corresponding to the "change" or "create" level. The cursor line can be moved with the (soft) cursor control keys.

Proposal 2: In this proposal the two monitors are not equipped with touch screens but their lowest line is reserved for a row of softkey labels which are operated by means of a row of keys below the screens. Thus in this proposal the two monitors are equipped with two rows of keys: one row of function keys and one row of softkeys. The meaning of the softkey labels depends on the level in the command tree. In Fig. 6.5 a possible key arrangement for the graph display is presented.

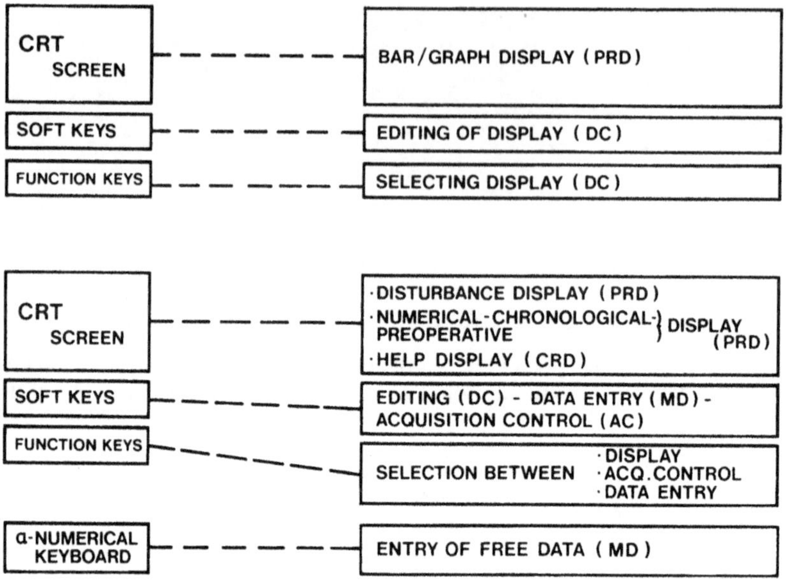

Fig. 6.6 To improve man-machine interaction the two color monitors can both be equipped with a row of softkeys and a row of function keys (left). This way commands can be entered at the screen in question. The communication which takes place via each of the devices is given on the right of the figure. The abbreviations stem from Fig. 6.2 and indicate the character of the interaction.

Conclusions: The first proposal is somewhat more sophisticated than the second and enables manipulation techniques. However, some more experience with a touch screen in the OR is desirable before this proposal is realized. For the moment we favor the second proposal. It is potentially cheaper and not necessarily a less agreeable solution. In Fig. 6.6 a schematic is given of the functions allotted to the input and output devices in the case of proposal 2.

The devices as discussed above may become outdated, but the underlying guidelines for selecting them will remain:

- A command set must be adjusted to the various types of users both experienced and inexperienced. In the OR environment there will be always a lack of time for interaction; operation of the system is a subordinate matter and attention must not be distracted away from the patient.
- The input devices must be adjusted to the command set but the number of different devices must be kept at a minimum while at the same time entering of all types of commands must be easy.
- Some flexibility must be guaranteed to enable small changes in the software.
- The interaction protocol may be a combination of all different principles as long as a logical and easy use is guaranteed.

6.3 Ergonomics: Information Presentation

In the previous section, proposals which focused on improved man-machine interaction were discussed. In this section we shall discuss some aspects of information presentation: the requirements for the legibility of (a series of) characters and the use of color.

6.3.1 Legibility

An image on a CRT screen is formed by three electron beams which scan the screen with a high frequency. Each beam illuminates either red-, blue- or green-colored phosphor pixels. Depending on the intensity relations of the illuminating beams, dots in different colors can result.

The quality of the symbols composed of these colored dots depends on many factors:

1. hardware properties of the screen such as the distance between the dots, the frame repetition rate, the focusing of the electron beam, etc.
2. the luminance of the screen, the illuminance from the surroundings, diffuse and specular reflection and the contrast of the characters.
3. the properties of the character set.

ad 1: Currently so-called high-resolution screens are available. These meet most requirements with respect to the points mentioned under 1. Their frame repetition rate is 50 Hz or more.

ad 2: Leebeek (1980) gives most of the necessary information on this point. The luminance of fields/information on CRT screens is mostly between 50 and 200 cd/m^2. The contrast between text and background is not only dependent on the basic contrast between the characters and the background which can be realized with the intrinsic luminance of the screen, but also on the light coming from the environment which is diffusely reflected by the screen. For normal circumstances Leebeek recommends illumination values of the work space ranging from 250-750 lux (100 lux => 30 cd/m^2 if 100% diffusely reflected). For the surgical work in the OR this value must be higher. Oborne (1985 p198) gives a table in which the type of work is listed against the required illumination of the workplace: for minute work an illumination of 3000 lux is mentioned. Pütsep (1979) even prescribes values of 40,000 lux at the plane of incision; of course, this value will be lower at the monitoring equipment.

Depending on the illumination and the reflection factor of the screen, the contrast on the screen will be decreased. Diffuse reflection factors may range from 0.05 to 0.30 and it is recommended in principle, for light characters on a dark background, that the contrast [defined as the luminance ratio between information (Li) and background (Lb)] be between 5 and 15, while contrasts between 7 and 12 are favored (advice on this aspect differs; for a review see Oborne 1985, p200). The Dutch *arbeidsinspectie* (1979, p29) presents a table in which the desired amount of light on the screen (basic luminance plus diffuse reflected luminance) is given as a function of text luminance and reflection factor. For instance, to obtain a luminance ratio between 5 and 15 when the text luminance is 150 cd/m^2 and the reflection factor is 0.10, the desired illuminance at the screen must be in the range of 300-900 lux.

Apart from the diffuse reflection, the specular reflection may influence legibility of the information. While diffuse reflection is not disadvantageous as long as it is included in the setting of the luminance ratio, specular reflection is always disturbing. It means that a specific light source is reflected at the transition from air to screen. Reflection causes the screen user to focus involuntarily on the reflected image; the corresponding superfluous accommodative movements can speed up fatigue. Apart from this the luminance ratio on the screen is locally diminished. Generally, it is required that the luminance of a reflected image be less than 10% of the luminance of the information on the screen. The luminance of the reflected image depends on the luminance of the reflected object and the so-called specular reflection factor of the screen surface following $L_{refl} = L_{obj} \cdot r_{refl}$, wherein for standard screens $r_{refl} = 4\%$ (when looking at the screen from a right angle). The best way to reduce reflection is by application of a coating on the screen surface; this reduces r_{refl} to 0.5%. A simple solution is to take care of indirect lighting by the screening of fluorescent lamps and windows, a measure which is strongly recommended.

Apart from these guidelines concerning the contrast of the information on the screen, guidelines are given with respect to the mean luminance of a display in relation to its environment in order to minimize adaptation effort. It is recommended that the increase in contrast from directly observed (low luminance) space to other parts of the visual field be gradual, with steps of minimally 3 and a maximal total contrast quotient of 10. This guideline gives reason to think that a light screen background is better than a dark background. An example: a screen with a mean intrinsic luminance of 100 cd/m^2 and a reflection factor of 0.30 is illuminated by a surrounding with a luminance of 3000 cd/m^2. Then it can be derived that the luminance at the screen is 1000 cd/m^2. Because of the considerable reflection, a sufficient contrast ratio of 3 between screen and direct surround is reached; with lower reflection factors a higher intrinsic screen luminance would be required.

From investigations by Radl (1980) and Bauer and Cavonius (1980) it followed that indeed a light background with dark characters (negative contrast) significantly enhances legibility. Moreover, Bauer et al. (1981) described the positive influence of a light background on specular reflection, although they also showed that a disadvantage of a light background is that flicker is more easily observed (Bauer et al. 1983). They determined that, if 95% of their population should not observe flicker on a CRT screen with a mean luminance of 80 cd/m^2, a frame repetition rate of 87 Hz was required. This is a much higher value than that found in standard studies on the so-called critical flicker frequency.

ad 3: The quantities relevant for the legibility of a character or strings of characters are defined in Fig. 6.7.

Coolen (1985) obtained the requirements for these quantities mainly using the work of Brauninger (1983), who performed a detailed literature study on this sub-

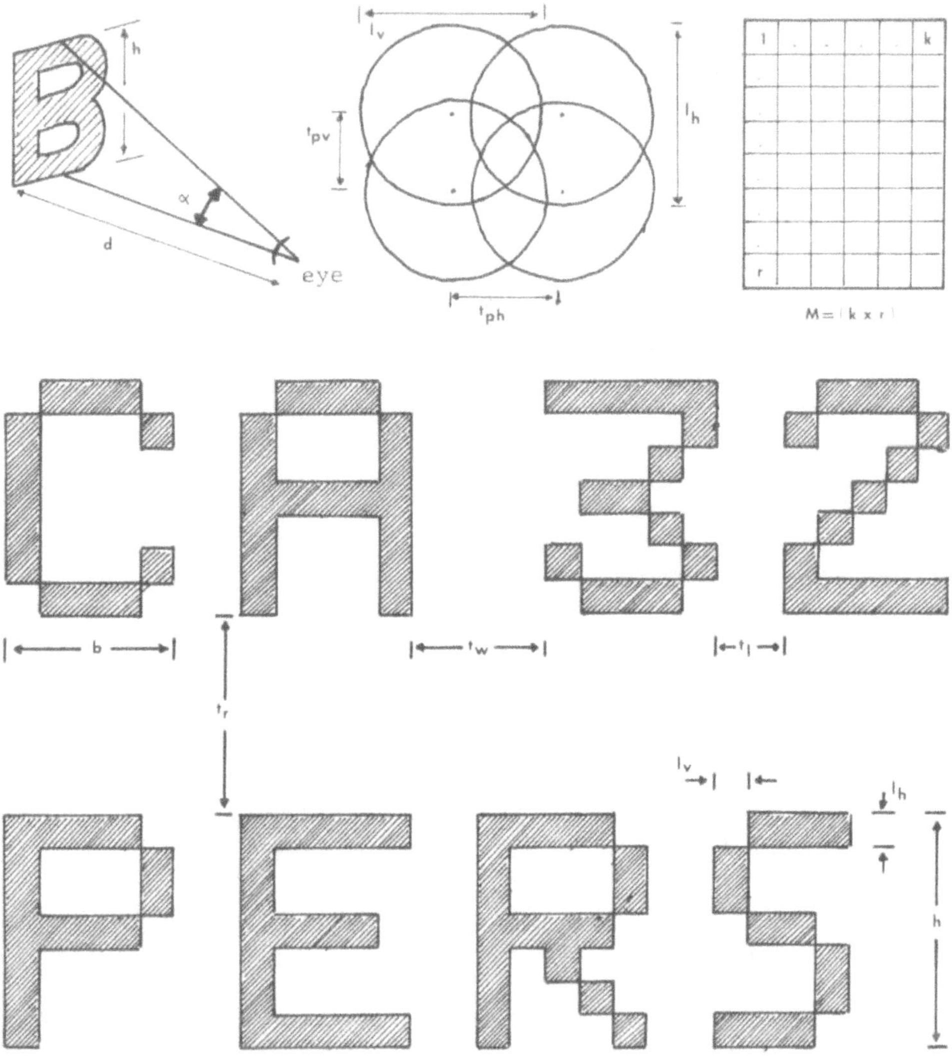

Fig. 6.7 To warrant optimal legibility of characters (and symbols), the dimensions of and between the characters must meet certain requirements. The relevant parameters are presented in the figure:

d	: viewing distance	l_h	: line width horizontal line
h	: character height	l_v	: line width vertical line
α	: visual angle h/d	t_{ph}	: horizontal dot distance
t_l	: character interspace	t_{pv}	: vertical dot distance
t_w	: word interspace	k	: number of dots in character matrix (horizontally)
t_r	: line interspace	r	: number of dots in character matrix (vertically)
b	: character width	M	: dimension of character matrix (k · r)

ject. The size of the observed object must be minimally 1/150 of the viewing distance (which corresponds with a viewing angle of at least 22°) with a minimum character size of 3 mm.

Leebeek (1980) recommends that the dots of which the characters are composed have sharp boundaries and Brauninger (1983) states that the dots must be round or square and that oval shapes must be avoided. The other requirements are listed

Table 6.2 The requirements for the parameters which determine the legibility of the characters †

$\frac{b}{h}$	70–100%					G
	50– 70%					S
	40– 50%					I
	0– 40%					B
$\frac{l_{h,v}}{h}$	7– 20%					G
$\frac{t_l}{h}$	*** > 7%	$\frac{t_l}{b}$	> 20%	$\frac{t_l}{l}$	> 100%	G
	6– 7%		10–20%		50–100%	S
	< 6%		< 10%		< 50%	I
$\frac{t_r}{h}$	> 100%					G
	80–100%					S
	50– 80%					I
	< 50%					B
$\frac{t_w}{h}$	75–100%					R*
$\frac{t_{ph}}{l_v}$ and $\frac{t_{ph}}{l_h}$	< 75%			$\left\lvert\frac{t_{ph}}{l_h}-\frac{t_{ph}}{l_v}\right\rvert$	< 20%	G
	75–100%				20–40%	S
	100–150%				40–60%	I
	> 150%				> 60%	B
M capitals	(Lincoln Mitre) 7×9	G				
	5×7					
	6×9	S				
	7×7					
	4×7	I				
	** (IPO normal incl. surround) 12×10	G			G good S sufficient I insufficient B bad R recommended	

† The symbols refer to the definitions given in Fig. 6.7.
* This range is as advised by Den Buurman (1977).
**The IPO normal set is a complete alphanumeric set with both upper and lower case characters (van Nes 1983). Note: these requirements were in fact collected for light characters on a dark background.
***It seems strange that distinction such as between > 7% (good) and 6–7% for t_l/h (sufficient) is made.

in Table 6.2. These are expressed in relation to the character height and rated from good to bad.

We applied these criteria to the new DADS high resolution screens. The results of the measurements are given in Table 6.3. The results hold for a reading distance of 0.64–0.81 m.

From Table 6.3 it can be concluded that:

- The character size is insufficient for viewing distances of more than one meter.
- Line interspacing is bad.
- The ratio between vertical dot distance and horizontal line width is insufficient: the vertical lines are dotted.
- The shape and the matrix dimension of the characters could be better.
- The remaining characteristics are sufficient or good. Coolen (1985) considered some measures to improve the disadvantageous properties. These included an increased line interspacing, an increase of character height, and the introduction of two character sizes. All measures result in a considerable decrease in the number of characters which can be presented on the display. Thus only the most urgent measures which have the most effect can be applied. Coolen determined that it is worth while to increase the line interspacing (this was implemented) and that the introduction of a second, bigger character size must be tried. Such a bigger character size would be applicable for presenting very important information such as alarm messages.

6.3.2 *Use and Function of Colors*

This subsection deals with the use and function of color (including black and white) so that it can be employed to achieve an optimal effect on readability (see for definitions of readability and legibility McCormick and Sanders 1983, p89). We shall check the colors currently employed in DADS as to their suitability and,

Table 6.3 The qualification of the information presentation on a high resolution screen

Parameter	Absolute measure	Relative measure	Qualification
h	4.7 mm	–	good
b	2.4 mm	$b/h = 51\%$	sufficient
l_h	0.6 mm	$l_h/h = 13\%$	good
l_v	0.5 mm	$l_v/h = 11\%$	good
t_l	1.0 mm	$t_l/h = 21\%$	good
		$t_l/b = 42\%$	good
		$t_l/l > 150\%$	good
t_w	4.3 mm	$t_w/h = 91\%$	sufficient
t_r	2.0 mm	$t_r/h = 43\%$	bad
t_{ph}	0.48 mm	$t_{ph}/l_v \cong 96\%$	sufficient
t_{pv}	0.67 mm	$t_{pv}/l_h \cong 112\%$	insufficient
$\lvert t_{ph}/l_v - t_{pv}/l_h \rvert$	16%	–	good
shape	slightly oval shaped	–	sufficient
M	5 × 7	–	sufficient

when necessary, suggestions for improvements will be made. It must be noted that the suggestions given in this section do not take all the fundamental properties of colors into account.

When colors are applied we have to deal with two types of contrast: luminance contrast and color contrast. The readability of colored information on a colored background depends on both.

The luminance of a color is often expressed in its luminance relative to white. The colors on CRT screens are composed by the illumination of red, green and blue phosphors with the property that the resulting color is formed according to:

$$L_{rel} = 0.30 \cdot R + 0.59 \cdot G + 0.11 \cdot B$$

Usually the intensity of the electron beams illuminating these basic colors is either on (1) or off (0) and the standard colors which are used on almost every CRT screen are composed in this manner. These include black, blue, green, cyan, red, magenta, yellow, and white, each with a fixed relative luminance according to the formula above. However, all kinds of other colors can be obtained by choosing settings of the beam intensity between 0 and 1. To this end Coolen (1985) developed a circuit to enable control of the beam intensities between 0 and 1. The question now is which combinations of fore- and background colors provide the best readability. There are three papers describing experiments for determining the best combinations of the standard colors as appearing on CRT screens.

Bruce and Foster (1982) made a selection based on the recognition time for a character; Colin (1983) measured the number of correctly read characters and Murch (1984) determined the preference of the users.

From their results we extracted an average judgement regarding color combinations both for dark characters on a light background and the reverse. This average qualification is presented in Table 6.4.

Table 6.4 The average qualification of color on color information as derived from three different investigations

Background / Foreground	White	Yellow	Cyan	Green	Magenta	Red	Blue	Black
White	–	–	–	±	+	+	+	+
Yellow	–	–	–	–	±	+	+	+
Cyan	±	–	–	–	–	±	+	+
Green	±	±	–	–	±	±	–	+
Magenta	±	±	±	±	–	–	±	±
Red	+	+	+	+	–	–	±	±
Blue	+	+	+	+	±	–	–	–
Black	+	+	+	+	+	+	–	–

– bad, ± moderate, + good

It is interesting to compare this qualification with that which can be obtained by judging the color combinations exclusively on their luminance ratio. We mentioned in the previous section that, for black-and-white information the acceptable range for this contrast is between 5 and 15. In Table 6.5 the luminance ratio for every combination of standard colors is given. When we judge the combinations on their ratio we find that only combinations of white, yellow, cyan, and green with black or blue are acceptable. Thus this method of judging provides fewer acceptable combinations than the performance tests as done by Bruce and Foster, Colin, and Murch. However, when we expand the acceptable ratio to between 2 and 3 (a range which can also be found in literature) the corresponding combinations increase (Table 6.6).

Table 6.5 Luminance ratios for standard colors

Background / Foreground	White	Yellow	Cyan	Green	Magenta	Red	Blue	Black
White	1.0	1.1	1.4	1.7	2.4	3.3	9.1	>
Yellow	1.1	1.0	1.3	1.5	2.2	3.0	8.1	>
Cyan	1.4	1.3	1.0	1.2	1.7	2.3	6.4	>
Green	1.7	1.5	1.2	1.0	1.4	2.0	5.4	>
Magenta	2.4	2.2	1.7	1.4	1.0	1.4	3.7	>
Red	3.3	3.0	2.3	2.0	1.4	1.0	2.7	>
Blue	9.1	8.1	6.4	5.4	3.7	2.7	1.0	>
Black	>	>	>	>	>	>	>	1

Table 6.6 Qualification of color combinations based on their luminance ratio (>2)

Background / Foreground	White	Yellow	Cyan	Green	Magenta	Red	Blue	Black
White	–	–	–	–	±	+	+	+
Yellow	–	–	–	–	±	+	+	+
Cyan	–	–	–	–	–	±	+	+
Green	–	–	–	–	–	±	+	+
Magenta	±	±	–	–	–	–	+	+
Red	+	+	±	±	–	–	±	±
Blue	+	+	+	+	+	±	–	±
Black	+	+	+	+	+	±	±	–

We find, then, that the judgement of color combinations on luminance alone agrees on relatively few combinations with the judgement on both luminance and color contrast as given in Table 6.4. The cause of this may lie in a dominant luminance component in the tested color combinations. Until further research has been performed, we recommend the use of standard color combinations which have been judged as acceptable according to Table 6.4.

This resulted in:

good combinations (light characters on dark background)	white on magenta,red,blue,black yellow on red,blue,black cyan on blue,black green on black
good combinations (dark characters on light background)	black on white,yellow,cyan,green, magenta,red blue on white,yellow,cyan,green red on white,yellow,cyan,green

The combinations which were given regard the use of two colors. When more colors are needed, we shall solve dilemmas by means of the guidelines for color coding which will be discussed later on.

As stated above, the combinations as judged to be acceptable in Tables 6.4 and 6.6 show a rather strong correspondence. Therefore, although it is a simplification, we shall in the following use the luminance ratio to judge the suitability of non-standard colors in case these seem necessary to improve the use of color in DADS.

In general, *when* more than one color is used for data presentation on a screen, the colors have a specific meaning : that is, the color is used to enhance the information to be presented. For instance, red is often used for alarms, or every element within a colored frame belongs to a single aspect of the presented information.

This is called color coding. Coolen (1985) and Buys (1985) derived the following guidelines for color coding:

- The number of colors used must be limited from about 4 on text displays to 7 for a graphical display.
- The colors must have a clear function and superfluous use should be avoided.
- The luminance quotients should guarantee acceptable readability.
- The coding must be simple and consistent, i.e. it should not change in time and place.
- The coding must be simple and surveyable, i.e. there should not be too many categories and they must be easy to memorize, which is facilitated by making the colors correspond to their emotional value.
- The coding must be at least partially redundant (colorblindness may occur), implying that color should not be the only coding dimension.

Application of the Color Criteria on the Displays of DADS: Based on the requirements derived above, we checked whether the use of colors on the displays of DADS corresponds with these requirements, and where necessary, recommendations for improvement will be given.

The Graphical Display: The number of colors applied is correct, the luminance of the colors used for textual information is sufficient. The use of magenta for the rods does not belong to the best combinations.

The Bar Display: The number of applied colors is correct but their use is not always consistent with their emotional value. For instance, the (safe) norm zone is blue instead of green; the present value is in green while not necessarily at a safe level. The red of the alarm bands and also the blue of the norm bands are somewhat too conspicuous relative to the small white time plots.

The Numerical/Disturbance/Communication Display: The number of applied colors is rather high. Only the use of red on black to indicate bad processing does not conform with the luminance criteria. The use of two different colors for presenting time and text of a disturbance message is superfluous.

With a somewhat adjusted set of colors the use of color in *the bar and graphical displays* can be improved:

This set consists of 4 background and 4 foreground colors (Table 6.7), from which no more than 7 combinations are to be used in each display.

The modifications we suggest for the graphical display include blue for the rods and cyan for the lines of the plot of related variables.

In the bar display the new color set can be applied as presented in Fig. 6.8; The colors of the zones are less dominant and overall the use of color is more consistent.

For the *numeric/disturbance/communication display* an adjusted color set is also recommended (Table 6.8).

Only orange is different from the former color set. Orange can be used for the disturbances because it has a warning character. The neutral colors white and cyan are recommended for the communication display. The color for the numerical

Table 6.7 The adjusted set of color combinations for the graphical and the bar display with their relative luminances

Background / Foreground	White	Yellow	Cyan	Green	Darkgreen	Darkred	Blue	Black
White					+	+	+	+
Yellow					+	+	+	+
Cyan					+	+	+	+
Green					±	+	+	+
Darkgreen	+	+	+	±				
Darkred	+	+	+	+				
Blue	+	+	+	+				
Black	+	+	+	+				

Color	L_{rel}
White	1.00
Yellow	0.89
Cyan	0.70
Green	0.59
Darkgreen	0.20
Darkred	0.20
Blue	0.11
Black	0

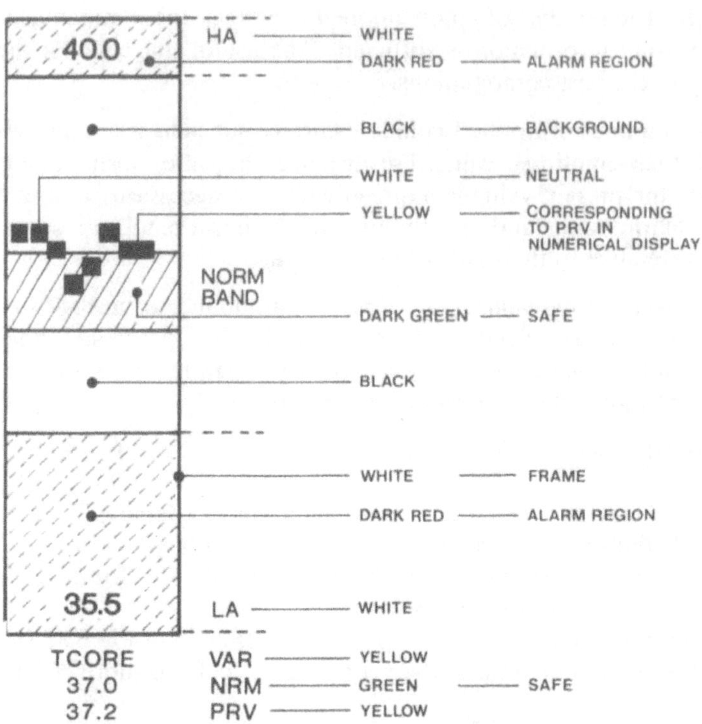

Fig. 6.8 The recommended colors for the bar display.

Table 6.8 The adjusted color set for the lower color monitor

Foreground \ Background	White	Yellow	Cyan	Orange	Red	Black
White					+	+
Yellow					+	+
Cyan						+
Orange						+
Red	+	+				
Black	+	+	+	+		

Color	L_{rel}
White	1.00
Yellow	0.89
Cyan	0.70
Orange	0.50
Red	0.30
Black	0

values is yellow, thus corresponding to the present values on the bar display. Yellow on red can be used to indicate transition of alarm limits. In this way the use of colors is kept at an essential minimum. The dark colors as advised for the bar display are not included: because of their low luminance they are not the most suitable for the detailed information on the numeric display.

6.4 DADS4: The Integrated Workstation

To obtain criteria for redesign of DADS, we mentioned in Chapter 2 the necessity of considering the whole operating team as it functions within the operating room. From those observations we derived the following conclusions:

- Optimal use of the facilities provided by DADS is only possible when DADS, just as the other monitoring equipment, is placed as near as possible to the head of the patient, within direct reach and vision of the anesthesiologist.
- To provide real centralized monitoring without groups of variables presented separately, all variables including respiratory values, cardiac output, and even clinical laboratory data, should be made available to DADS.
- To avoid the situation in which the anesthesiologist monitors respiration by means of DADS while being required to set the parameters on the ventilator, DADS and the relevant front-end equipment should be integrated in such a way that DADS can be used to set the desired values on the front-end equipment.
- Just before and during bypass and while weaning from bypass, transfer of information between the anesthesiologist and the perfusionist takes place. Thus automation with centralized display etc. should not only be available for the anesthesiologist but as far as useful also to other disciplines: data transfer should be improved.
- Efficient patient-monitoring can only be enhanced and is less prone to errors when more integration and uniformity is achieved and when equipment setup is according to human engineering standards.

Continuing on these lines and taking into account all the ideas for improving DADS, it was decided to start the design of an updated version of DADS (DADS4).

To this end a sequence of focused group discussions took place. Participating were engineers, physicians, and industrial partners. The phases completed were:

- Determination of the objectives of the new version and of the type of surgical and/or anesthetic procedure for which DADS4 should be designed
- Determination and mapping of basic components and facilities
- Finishing and perfecting of the design.

There are several objectives with which a new DADS can be designed; it is possible to use all the newest ideas and hardware devices in a design of a futuristic DADS. However, this will not result in a workable design for which the components are directly available. Another possibility is to design a manufacturable "top-of-the-line" prototype which must be tested prior to production, but such a prototype is not suitable for studying facilities which are as yet not marketable. Therefore it was decided to develop a compromise: a "maxi"-DADS, a feasible design which can be developed at a short notice, with optimal research capabilities and with flexibility for incorporating new ideas. Suitable algorithms, design criteria, principles of man-machine interaction, etc. would, in a later phase, be incorporated by the industrial partners into a manufacturable product.

The *design* of DADS4 would again be directed toward complex surgical and anesthetic procedures: cardiac surgery, neurosurgery, transplantations, orthopaedic surgery, and major vessel surgery.

Farrow et al. (1984) selected 9 types of surgery on their mortality rate: fractures, larynx and trachea, laparotomy, amputation, open heart, oesophagus, colon and rectum, joints, and upper gastrointestinal tract.

These last procedures are not necessarily the most complex, but might be those where prevention of critical incidents by means of advanced monitoring has the greatest impact. At this stage the value of DADS for high-risk patients (high ASA score) or young, healthy patients has not been discussed.

Based on the conclusions from the beginning of this section regarding the position of DADS and the required central operation of all equipment, the major requirement for DADS4 is that the ventilator must be part of the design. This is already common usage at simpler surgical procedures, where ventilation and monitoring equipment are placed on or around one cart. Also, both Boquet (1980) and Cooper et al. (1978) combined ventilation and monitoring in their design of a new anesthesia delivery system. In designing an anesthesia delivery/monitoring workstation, De Roo (1980) investigated position changes of the anesthesiologist with respect to his equipment; he concludes: "Many changes in position of the anesthesiologists can be prevented when integration of anesthesia delivery and monitoring equipment is realized."

Apart from the ventilator, more devices are placed very close to the patient for reasons of frequency of use, ease of reach etc. Therefore, apart from the ventilator, the capnograph and the cardiac output computer will also be included in the design and, if possible, the O_2 analyzer, a noninvasive blood pressure monitor and an analyzer for the activated clotting time.

The specific DADS4 components will consist of:

- A monitor (with softkeys) for presentation of the bar and graph displays (14-in.)
- A monitor (with softkeys) for presentation of the numerical, medical data and disturbance information (14-in.)
- And, replacing the CRT screen in the main conventional monitoring rack, a third additional monitor (with softkeys) for displaying the analogue signals (12 or 14-in.). This is a first step toward the incorporation of the hemodynamic monitoring equipment into DADS.
- An event pad. On the previous version of DADS one event-key was implemented for fast marking of clinically significant events, but event entry is still not optimal. In the case of a few sequential events, it becomes troublesome to memorize which event number corresponds to which event, and there is a reasonable chance that entry of some events will be forgotten. Therefore, an event pad based on ideas presented by Ornato et al. (1981) is in preparation.
- A keyboard for the remaining interaction.
- 2 Floppy drives for storage and retrieval of programs and data.
- The electronic components (processors, memory boards, power systems).

In DADS4 all essential information should be presented on the screens. Therefore it is likely that the plotter for generation of the anesthesia record will not be required in direct proximity to the anesthesia equipment. Positioning in a corner or directly outside the OR seems useful.

The hardware devices to be included in DADS4 are mentioned above. At this stage it is not possible to anticipate all the requirements regarding software specifications. However, the improvements suggested for the man-machine interaction (Section 6.2) and the data presentation (Section 6.3) will be implemented. The event pad will require additional software, as will the presentation of analogue signals. Moreover, a new algorithm for the detection of disturbances will be implemented (Blom et al. 1985, Meijler and Beneken 1986).

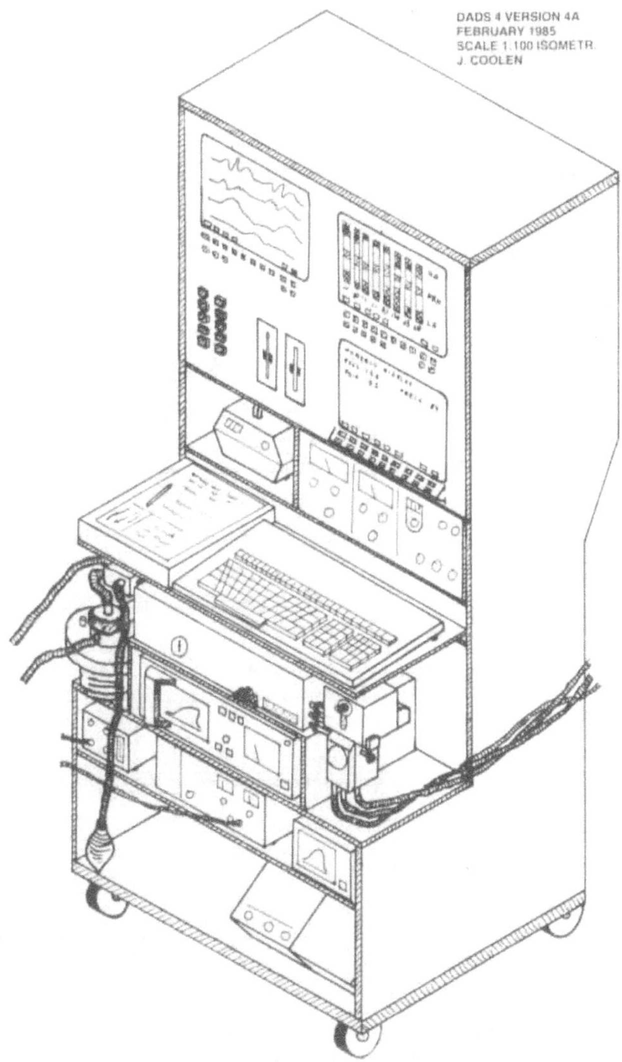

Fig. 6.9 The final design for the DADS4 system. Its main property is that it integrates all the various devices to be used by the anesthesiologist in monitoring. It is a first step toward "cockpit"-based monitoring.

After three intermediate drafts, a final design was completed (Figs. 6.9 and 6.10). Some specifics about the design:

- Protruding parts such as tubes and knobs belonging to the humidifier, the vaporizer, and the ventilator had to be incorporated. It is essential that these devices be accessible. Among other things, it must be possible to change tubes and to refill the vaporizers.
- A special problem was the location of the ventilator. At first the ventilator was planned below the keyboard. However, as long as control of the ventilator does not take place via DADS, this would mean that the positioning of this critical control would be too low and does not meet ergonomic requirements. To solve this, it was decided to place the electronic part of the ventilator (the part with

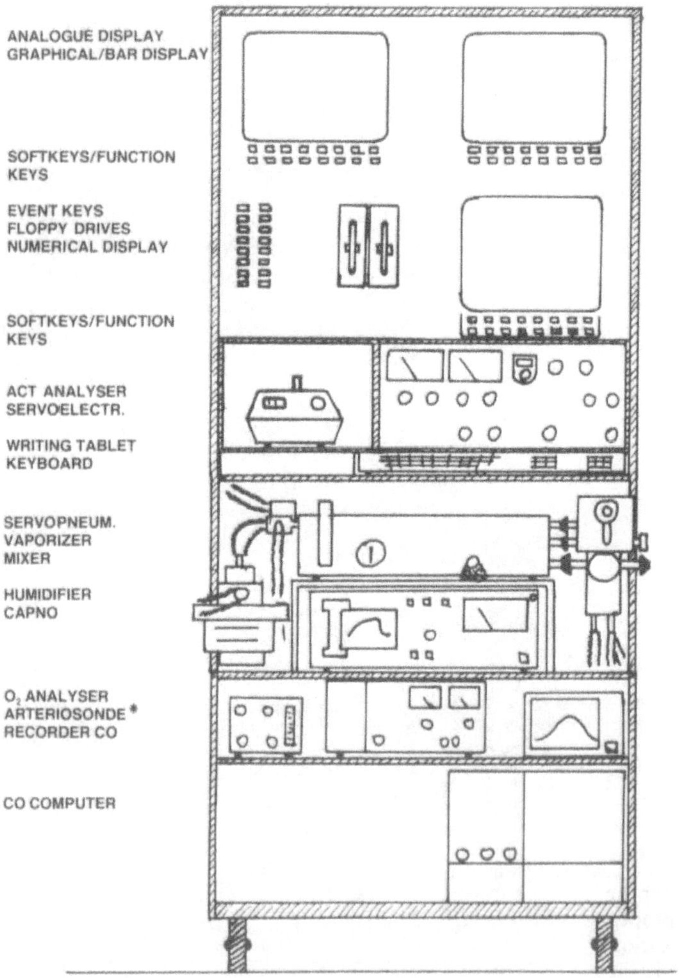

Fig. 6.10 The front view of DADS4. * Arteriosonde stands for a noninvasive, ultrasound based blood pressure measuring device.

the controls) just above the keyboard. The pneumatic part of the ventilator remained below the keyboard to prevent cluttering of the upper part of DADS4. In case of failures, this pneumatic part must be quickly and easily accessible from above; to enable this, the entire panel with keyboard and writing tablet was fixed onto a drawer which can be pushed inward.
- The location of the electronic part of the ventilator influenced the overall impression of DADS4. The central part of the setup was designed as a standard on which the upper and wider part of DADS4 with the monitors could rest. With the ventilator, the central part had to be made as wide as the upper part, thus giving the design a heavier appearance than planned. It had also been planned to place the lower monitor at a small angle with the vertical plane to ensure an optimal viewing angle for this lower monitor from the standing position of the anesthesiologist, but because this would obscure the view on the ventilator controls, this idea had to be discarded as well.

Discussion of the Design: The dimensions and composition of DADS4 were primarily determined by the devices to be included and the physical circumstances in the operating room. This implies that compromises had to be made between human engineering requirements and feasibility. Below we shall check the ultimate setup of DADS4 in two ways:

1. The vertical positioning of the main components of DADS against the absolute measures which were derived from literature.
2. The relative positioning of the components in the entire setup.

ad 1: Table 6.9 shows the qualification of the vertical positioning of the main components of DADS4, based on guidelines as derived from Dreyfuss (1967) for consoles and panels applied in the office and in control rooms.

From Table 6.9 it can be seen that the absolute height of most components is satisfactory, but that some components are positioned somewhat too low.

ad 2: Döring (1976b) describes the techniques applied to the design of cockpits in aircraft. In order to place every component at its optimal position, the devices are

Table 6.9 The qualification of the height of the main components of DADS4

Component		height	judgement
Displays	analogue	150-170 cm	good
	bar/graph	150-170 cm	good
	numerical	120-140 cm	moderate
Controls	function/soft-keys analogue	145-155 cm	good
	function/soft-keys bar/graph	145-155 cm	good
	function/soft-keys numerical	115-125 cm	sufficient
	ventilator	105 cm	moderate
	keyboard	90 cm	sufficient
	writing pad	95 cm	moderate

rated with respect to a number of requirements (McCormick and Sanders 1983, p343) such as frequency of use, criticality of use, etc. From the resulting tables component positions can be derived; below we will apply this technique to check the placement of the DADS4 components. To this end, the components incorporated in the system were rated on their importance for:

- the efficiency and efficacy of the control and monitoring task of the anesthesiologist (IMP) (high, medium, low)
- their frequency of use by the anesthesiologist (FREQ) (high, medium, low)
- the duration of one action of the anesthesiologist at the device (TDUR) (continuous,extensive,brief)
- the critical value of the device for the immediate wellbeing of the patient (CRIT) (high, medium, low).

We judged the design of DADS4 on these criteria with respect to the required distance from the patient because of tubes, connections, etc., expressed in terms of the overall width of the system (DIST) (close, middle, far). Table 6.10 shows the resulting qualification.

The overall impression we get from this table is that the relative positioning of the devices is satisfactory. A problem can be expected in the control of the CO computer. In fact, all equipment positioned below the keyboard is unsuitable for operation and display. However, the display functions of most of these components will be taken over by DADS4 and their frequency of operation is low. In view of the desire for integration and positioning near the patient, no alternatives were possible.

At a later stage it can be expected that the systems which take care of integration will become smaller. It may be desirable that control and readout of the most important functions can take place on a screen that swings out close to the patient's head.

6.5 Summary

In this chapter we worked at ergonomic guidelines concerning three aspects of DADS, including man-machine interaction, information presentation, and layout of anesthesia equipment. When a selection of devices and protocols for man-machine interaction has to be made, the following rules must be kept in mind:

- The interaction must be easy both for experienced and inexperienced users.
- It must be virtually self-learning.
- Not the system but the patient needs and should receive attention.
- Some flexibility must be provided to enable minor changes in the interaction.
- The number of different devices for interaction must be kept at a minimum, but at the same time easy entry of the various inputs must be guaranteed.
- As long as it is logical, the interaction protocol may be a combination of several principles.

When departing from CRTs for data presentation, currently the touch-screen, soft- and function keys, and the conventional keyboard are the most suitable devices

Table 6.10 The qualification of the relative positioning of the components of DADS4

FUNCTION						
Monitor and control patient	IMP	FREQ	TDUR	CRIT	DIST	JUDGEMENT
Analogue display	H	H	B-E	H	F	satisfactory
Bar/Graph display	H	H	M	L	F	satisfactory
Numerical display	M	M	M	H	M	satisfactory
Event pad	H	H	B	M/L	C	satisfactory
Floppy drives	H	L	B	L	F	distance could have been greater
CO computer control part	M	M	E	M	C	probably too difficult to reach, unless with remote control
Electronic part ventilator	H	M	B	H	M	satisfactory
Keyboard	L	L	E	L	M	satisfactory
Writing pad	L	L	E	L	M	satisfactory
Humidifier	L	L	B	M	C	satisfactory
Vaporizer	L	L	E	H	F	access could be better
Mixer	L	L	B	H	F	satisfactory
Pneumatic part of ventilator	M	L	B-E	H	M	satisfactory
Capnograph	M	M	B	H	C	too low but hopefully monitoring functions can be performed by DADS components
O2 analyzer	H	L	B	M	C	idem
Noninvasive	M	L	M	M	C	satisfactory
ACT meter	H	H	B	L	F	rather low but mistakes are easily recognized

for interaction. However, this may change with new technical developments. In particular, the number of medical data which as yet cannot be automatically sampled and processed is considerable. This number may be reduced when progress in automation is further introduced into hospitals.

The study of guidelines on information presentation taught us that it is not self-evident that a high-resolution color screen guarantees optimal readability. When a new screen is bought, the properties of the default character set must be checked and, where necessary and possible, improved. Items such as line distance, word distance and matrix size must be checked , but also the intrinsic sizes of the character such as width relative to height must be sufficient.

The use of color can be very meaningful in enabling enhanced presentation of information by means of color coding. No more than 4–7 combinations must be applied. There are 23 acceptable combinations of standard colors in which, on the average, dark characters on a light background are somewhat more favored than light characters on a dark background.

If nonstandard colors are applied, it was derived that their luminance ratio must be at least 2. For DADS non standard colors such as orange, dark green, and dark red were introduced.

The arrangement of the work space of the anesthesiologist should be done in the same way as for an airplane cockpit. The following objectives must be pursued: integration, uniformity, uncluttering, comprehensiveness, and positioning in accordance to priority rules. Priority rules include: the importance for the control task of the anesthesiologist, the frequency of use, the task duration of one action at the device and the critical value of the device for the immediate wellbeing of the patient. These criteria have to be judged against the required distance of the component from the patient because of tubes and the like.

If these guidelines are followed, an integrated workstation can result which is less prone to mishaps than the current mixture of devices. Moreover, when a modular setup is supplied, the workstation can be stripped down or extended to be applicable in many different procedures.

7 The Automated Anesthesia Record

7.1 Introduction

In Section 2.4 it was shown that record keeping takes up about 12% of the time of the anesthesiologist. Apart from this, as will be illustrated below, there are considerable disadvantages in the use of handwritten records. Based on these considerations, this chapter will deal with the design and evaluation of an automated anesthesia record. The importance of realizing such a record was one of the outcomes from the evaluation procedure.

History: Because they wished to improve their technique of administering ether, Cushing and Codman started around 1895 with the registration of heart rate and respiration on what they called ether cards Fig. 7.1 (Beecher 1940). Some years later, Cushing's "blood pressure chart" is already comparable with current records. It presents vertical plots based on five-minute measurements of heart rate, systolic

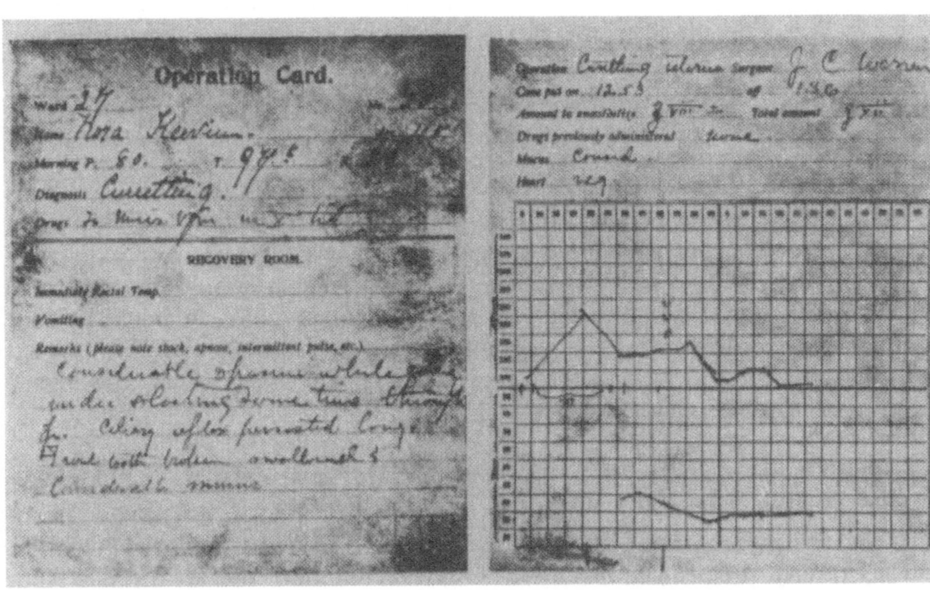

Fig. 7.1 The two sides of an early anesthesia record as used by Codman in 1894. (By permission of *Surgery, Gynecology and Obstetrics.*)

and diastolic arterial pressure, and of respiration. The most important events are written perpendicular to the plots at the corresponding time (Cushing 1903). Cushing writes that there are people voicing the opinion that over-elaborate records might take the administrator's mind off his primary task, but that he himself feels most emphatically that it keeps his mind on the task. He recommends keeping the old records for later: "Please put [these cards] in a corner of the Library, where some day some young fellow may brush the dust from them and say: 'Who were these fellows anyhow, and what is this "ether" they are talking about? Do you mean that people used to be put to sleep by the inhalation of drugs in the 19th century?" (Beecher 1940).

Since that time the records have become more complex, and record keeping is becoming more time-consuming with the increasing complexity of anesthetic procedures (Section 2.2). However, no essential changes have occurred in the principle of record keeping; much has been written about its value, the various methods, and the processing of the collected data. Hallen (1973) mentions the most important articles and Collins (1976) gives a concise survey. That there has not always been a uniform opinion regarding the need for record keeping can be illustrated by a rather unexpected question in an international examination paper for postgraduates (Mushin 1953):

The candidate had to indicate which answer was the correct one. "A well kept anesthesia record

a) demonstrates the artistic ability of the anesthesiologist;
b) helps the anesthesiologist to pass the time while squeezing the bag;
c) helps to support the paper industry;
d) by its very production contributes to the well-being of the patient; is an aid to the surgeon in his further care of the patient; helps the anesthesiologist in his evaluation of the drugs he uses, the techniques he employs, and the abilities and knowledge he has or does not have; and in a course such as this, is an obligation which each anesthesiologist has to his fellow trainees so that all may share to the fullest extent many more experiences in anesthesia than could be encountered on an individual basis in the same length of time".

Currently, the anesthesiologist is in fact obliged to make an anesthesia record for the provision of medicolegal documentation about the anesthetic procedure. However, from a questionnaire submitted to a large population of anesthesiologists in Great Britain and Ireland (Seed and Welsh 1976), it followed that 31.6% of anesthesiologists do not make records during minor operations and 23.8% regard it as a nuisance. As the reason for completing a record, 74.2% of the respondents mentioned the medicolegal aspect.

Functions: Beneken et al. (1983) and Schneider (1982) give the peri- and peroperative functions of the anesthesia record:

- Preoperatively: recording of demographic data, ASA score, diagnostic remarks, drug history, premedication, current physical condition, and appropriate laboratory values. These are then available peroperatively and can be used for planning the anesthesia management.

- Peroperatively: recording of type and volume of all fluids and blood products administered, dose and time of administration of anesthetic agents and other drugs, and other events occurring during the course of the operation, as well as the annotation of observations and signal values from the patient. This provides the legal evidence of monitoring during the procedure and enables the anesthesiologist to discover trends in signals and to evaluate the reaction to administered drugs and other interventions.
- Postoperatively: recording of the assessment of the patient's condition and transfer of information to the ICU. Other purposes are research, teaching, legal matters, and review prior to subsequent surgery.

Layout of the Anesthesia Records: Most records consist of the same types of component:

- Time-independent preoperative data, such as patient data, diagnostic remarks, etc.
- Time-independent peroperative data, for instance: size of the endotracheal tube, type of monitoring, etc.
- Lists with remarks and/or numerical data.
- Tables with special subsets of data as for instance blood gas values.
- Graphs/charts.

However, the arrangement of these components may differ strongly between layouts. Seed and Welsh (1976) give, derived from the questionnaires, a thorough review of the various types of record which are used. They found that varying sizes of charting space (from 5 · 10 cm to 10 · 15 cm) are used for graphical recording. In 82% of the records a blood pressure chart was available, and 53.9% had time scale spaces on the chart for recording the administered drugs. The most common arrangement (76.3%) was for the time scale to be on the horizontal axis and in 28.6% of the charts, symbols were suggested for the different parameters. A few of the records had a separate chart space for recording the concentration of inhalational agents given. A separate header and separate annotation space were available for:

- the induction (15.5%)
- airway management and intubation (32.0%)
- maintenance (21.4%)
- anesthetic techniques (26.7%)
- fluids (53.4%)
- notes/remarks (45.6%).

Problems with Handwritten Records: Irrespective of their layout, problems always occur with handwritten anesthesia records (Gravenstein 1980).

Legibility and Comprehensiveness: The legibility of handwriting is always a problem and even more so in the case of the anesthesia record, where data must often be entered in a hurry and mostly only a limited space on the record is available.

Completeness: One of the peroperative functions of the anesthesia record is to record monitored variables. Currently there are some guidelines as to what constitutes proper monitoring (Noback 1983, Gezondheidsraad 1982), but regulatory authorities do not specify the frequency with which vital signs should be measured. At present, intervals of five minutes are common clinical practice (Schneider 1982); however, mishaps resulting in permanent brain damage can occur within five minutes, while there are also cases in which the blood pressure varies little during the entire procedure. Another deficiency of the records is that they almost never show why a particular drug was given. Also, clinical observations such as those of the patient's color, responsiveness, etc. are almost never recorded.

Correctness: Record keeping takes about 12% of the anesthesiologist's time and normally does not present a problem. However, in moments of peak load, e.g. before and during induction, it is a problem. Zollinger et al. (1977) compared 100 cases of hand-recorded measurements of blood pressure with those obtained and plotted automatically. They noted that in many of these cases the physician did not begin to write until almost thirty minutes into the case, and it appeared that measurements were incompletely and inaccurately recorded. A similar study was performed by Whitesell et al. (priv. comm.). They also found that physiological data were more reliably recorded by the computerized monitoring system and that most discrepancies occurred during periods of maximum activity for the anesthesiologist. For the purpose of detecting differences in record-keeping of data which could not be sampled automatically, a study was performed by Baetz et al. (1979): two sets of twenty cases each were collected. For the cases in the first group an experienced nurse recorded the data as her only task, while the anesthesiologist, as usual, manually entered data in his record. For the second group control records were again kept by the nurse, and the anesthesiologists were able to use a so-called semiautomatic keypad. The record keeping of the anesthesiologists was compared with the "perfect" nurse-kept records. In the first group, of the 1379 required entries, 230 entries (17%) were missing, including 97 unrecorded blood pressure measurements, and 82 entries (6%) were incorrect in time or amount. In the second group, 1615 required entries were noted. Of these, 99 entries (6%) were missing, including 31 missed blood pressure entries. 137 entries (8%) were incorrect in time or amount. Again, the advantages of automation are clear.

7.2 The Automated Anesthesia Record

One of the important features of DADS is the centralized collection and storage of all data of interest during a procedure. This feature can be exploited by subsequently extracting these data for the automatic generation of an anesthesia record. This may reduce a number of the aforementioned problems. In summary, the advantages are:

- Reduction of the administrative workload, leaving more time for patient care.
- Improvement of the quality of the record because of objective and consistent recording (no rejection of "unusual" measuring values) and because of continuous recording also during critical periods, when the anesthesiologist needs to center his attention on the patient.

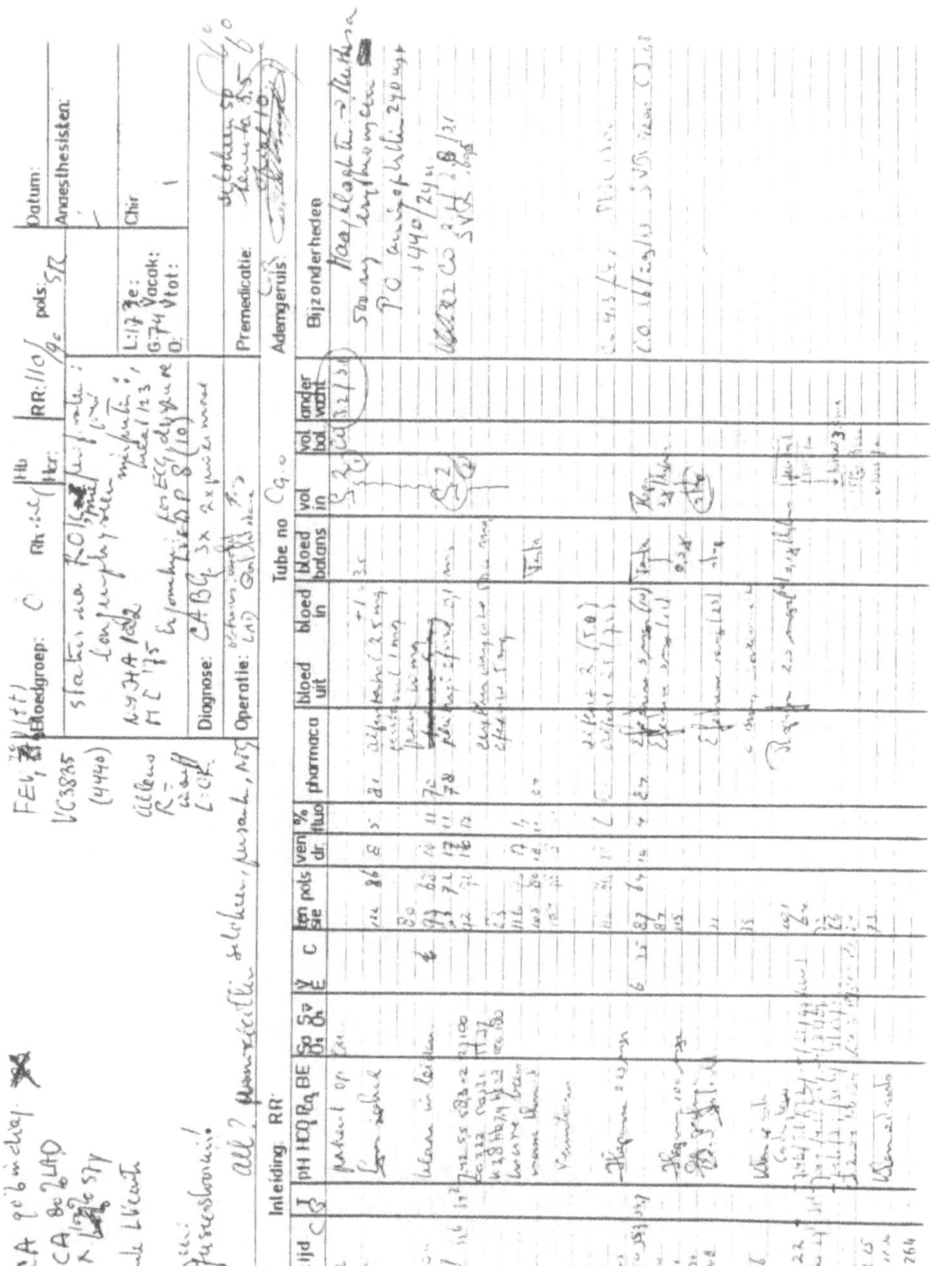

Fig. 7.2 A sample of a handwritten anesthesia record. The upper part contains demographic and preoperative data. In the lower part, printed headers and written information do not correspond. The recorded information contains from left to right: time, temperatures, interventions and values of blood gases and electrolytes, expired minute volume, CO_2ex, systolic and mean arterial pressure, diastolic pulmonary arterial pressure, right atrial pressure, heart rate, medications administered as a bolus and by means of an infusion, cardiac output values, miscellaneous values and comments.

- The machine-written record is more legible than the handwritten record, which is an advantage as the anesthesiologist is expected to make each and every record as if he were going to defend it in court (Schneider 1982).
- The machine-written record is flexible. Small changes can be easily realized.

Fig. 7.2 shows a handwritten record such as used during cardiac surgery at the University Hospital Leyden. The lack of legibility is obvious. It lacks graphical presentation of common variables such as blood pressures and heart rate. This is due to the fact that the anesthesiologists recognized the incompleteness and thus incorrectness of possible interpolations when putting the irregularly monitored variables into a graph. Furthermore, the layout of the record is outdated: headings and contents of columns no longer correspond.
Another problem is the discrepancy between the number of comments (irregularly entered medical data) and the interval recordings (regularly entered signal values). This prevents a definite correspondence between time of entry of comments and recorded data, and it is just this exact time correspondence which is so very important when it is necessary to retrace a procedure (Linnarsson 1985 priv. comm.).

To facilitate the introduction and acceptance of the automated record and enable switching to manual recording in case of problems, it was decided that the first design of an automated anesthesia record should be a "look-alike" of the handwritten record. This requires that the new list should consist of the standard record components (lists, graphs, tables, and the like) with an arrangement mainly in columns.

The design of the automated record coincided with the desire of the Leyden University Hospital, Department of Anesthesiology, to design a new record. Its design was accomplished after many detailed discussions between the anesthesiologists and the developers and has been described by van Kessel et al. (1986). It consists of two pages: a first page with preoperative information and possibly comments regarding the induction, and a second page for the peroperative data. Page 2 of a sample record is given in Fig. 7.3. In the centre are the graphs, including a time axis for continuous registration of automatically sampled blood pressures and heart rate. Heart rate (HR) and systemic arterial pressures (PSYS, MAP, PDIA) are plotted against the scale on the left (30->180 mmHg), mean pulmonary arterial pressure (MPAP) (and in most cases also the central venous pressure (MCVP)) is plotted in the scale at the right (-10->40 mmHg).

In order to provide the direct relation between comments and graphs, it was decided to draw the graphs in the vertical direction, with the comments perpendicular to them. The advantages of horizontal presentation of the comments and the definite relation between graphs and comments outweigh the possible disadvantages of vertical presentation of the graphs. To further enhance presentation in the graphs, four different colors are used for plotting the variables.

All text has a certain height, which, related to the time-axis, represents a certain duration of time (in our example 5 minutes). Thus, when many alphanumeric data are entered (more than one line per 5 minutes), the text columns will be filled before the graphs reach the end. To prevent a great discrepancy between the time axis of the graphs and the location of alphanumeric data, the alphanumeric columns are divided into two sections, each with its own time axis. To the left of the graphs, two columns are used for the administered drugs and the activated clotting time (ACT), because the ACT is directly related to the administered (anti)coagulant drugs. To the right of the graphs, one column is reserved to indicate start and stop of bypass and aorta-clamping. To the right of this column, and with a time scale corresponding to the far right axis, the remaining alphanumeric data are recorded in an order reflecting their relation to the blood pressure curves, from left to right: the cardiac output (which during bypass is the flow at the pump), the skin and core temperatures and the expiratory CO_2 concentration. The remaining columns can be used for other respiratory values and settings or fluid balance values. Thus, to prevent the readout of data without an exact time marking, the anesthesia record shows three time axes, one for the graphs and two for the alphanumeric data. The resolution of the graph time axis is fixed: in one graph 3.5 hours of data can be recorded. Thoracic procedures usually last about 6 hours, so two pages are necessary.

During generation of the anesthesia record, the time axes correspond as much as possible. This is achieved by placing the alphanumeric data as closely as possible to the corresponding time in the graphs, but never above this time; when only a few alphanumeric data are entered there will be empty lines in the corresponding columns.

When many alphanumeric data are entered the timeaxes may still show discrepancies because the timeaxis of the alphanumeric data runs ahead of the timeaxis on the graphs. However, in all situations exact times of all data can be extracted from the different timeaxes.

An extra facility is the entry of the events which are listed in Appendix 2.

When the special event key is pushed, the time is recorded and the word EVENT and a reference number are written in the comment column. Later on, the event can be explained by using the possibility of entering free comment referring to this reference number. The event marks are recorded immediately. The same holds for the entries made on the keyboard, such as free comment and event explanations. The signal values for the graphs are determined every 15 seconds and stored. Every 3 minutes the graphs are updated with the stored data. Continuously monitored, alphanumerically recorded signal values are updated every 10 minutes.

Apart from the central chart with graphs and alphanumerical data, two tables below this chart have been included: one for the presentation of blood gas values and electrolytes and one to plot the amount of administered (anti)coagulant drugs against the activated clotting time. The values can be plotted there as soon as they are automatically transferred to DADS and thus can be recognized by their own entry code. For the moment, they have to be entered as a comment by means of the keyboard.

7.3 Evaluation of the Automated Anesthesia Record

In the design of the automated record as described above, the guidelines for (re)design as given in Section 4.3, (such as knowledge retrieval, requirements definition and determination of alternatives) were followed. This resulted, within the conditions, in a reasonably optimal design; this was confirmed by the positive

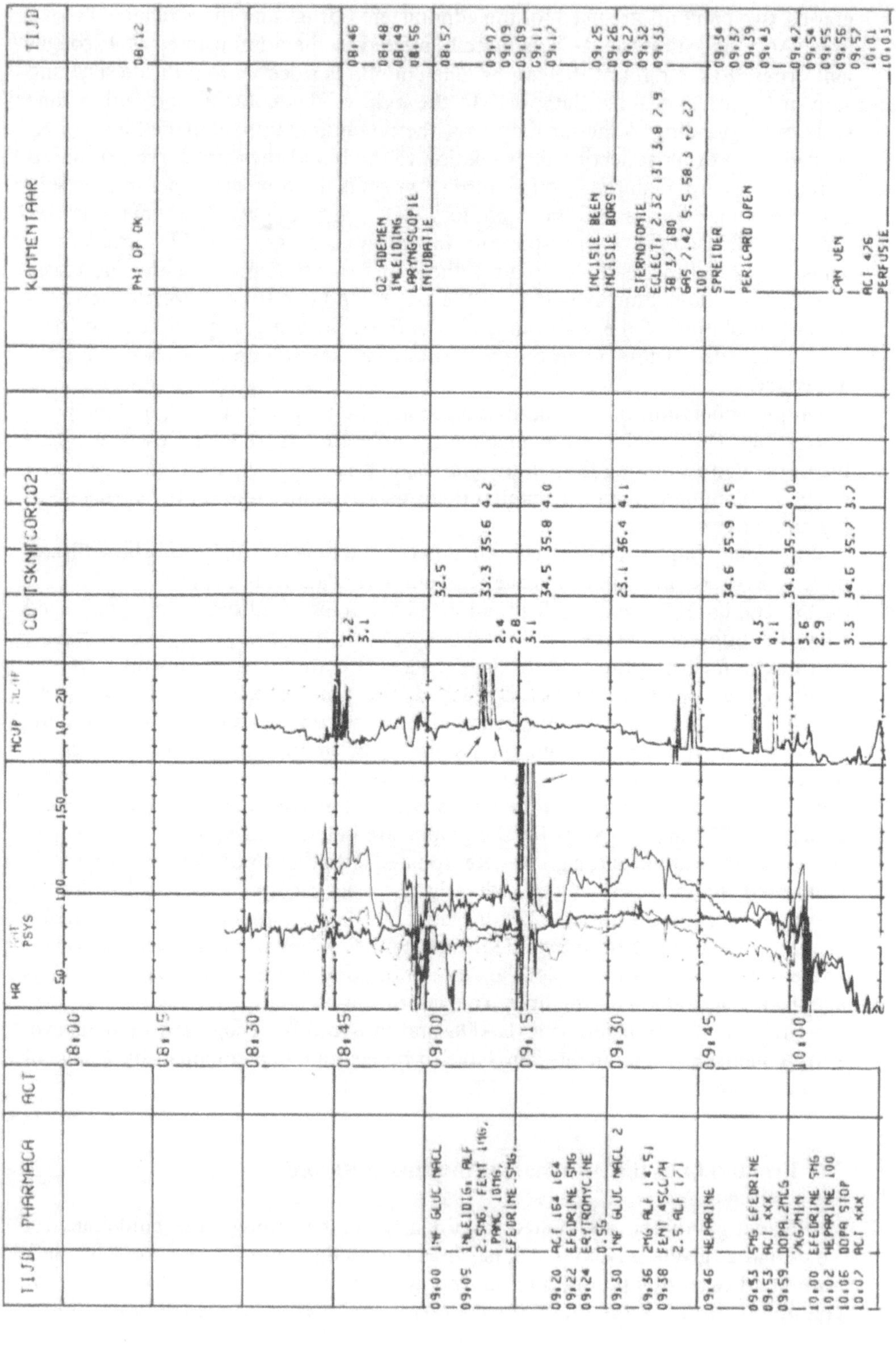
TIJD
PHARMACA
ACT
HR
PSYS
MCUP
CO
TSKN
TCOR
CO2
KOMMENTAAR
TIJD
08.00
08.15
08.30
08.45
09.00
09.15
09.30
09.45
10.00
PAT OP OK
O2 ADEMEN
INLEIDING
LARYNGSLOPIE
INTUBATIE
INCISIE BEEN
INCISIE BORST
STERNOTOMIE
SPREIDER
PERICARD OPEN
CAN VEN
PERFUSIE
INF GLUC NACL
HEPARINE
EFEDRINE
DOPA STOP

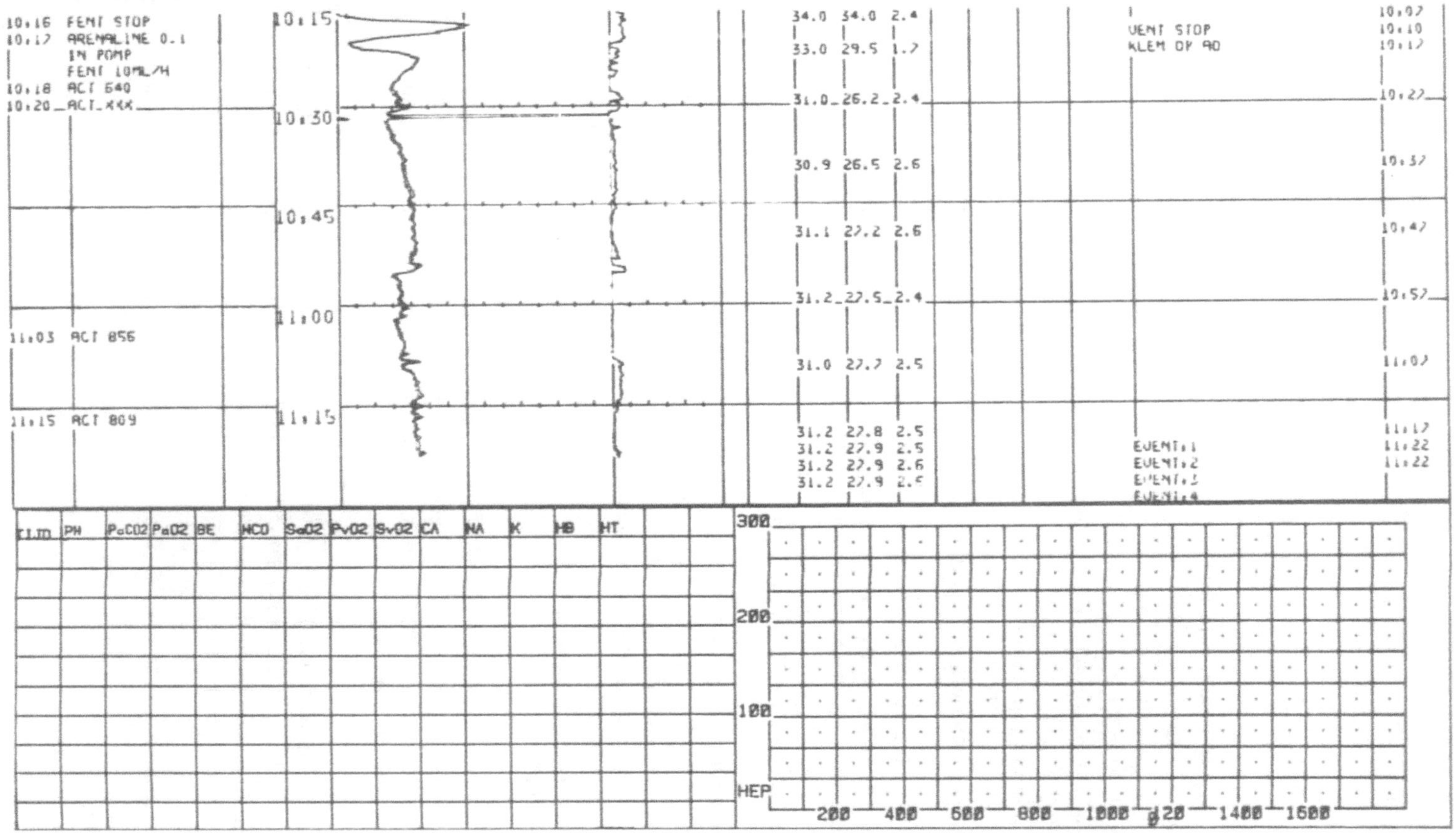

Fig. 7.3 A sample of Page 2 of an automated anesthesia record. The color information is lost in the printing process. The lower part of the record contains two tables: one for blood gas and electrolyte values and one for coagulation information. The main part shows, from left to right:

- 1st time axis, belonging to the next two columns
- column for administered drugs (bolus, perfusors and volatiles)
- column for activated clotting times
- 2nd time axis, belonging to the graphs
- graphs of heart rate and arterial pressures in the left range, graphs of mean central venous pressure, mean left atrial pressure and mean pulmonary arterial pressure in the right range

reactions from the users. However, we thought it useful to optimize the design based upon remarks made by a somewhat larger group of anesthesiologists and on practical experience with the record. To this end, a questionnaire was composed consisting of 9 open ended questions, 3 multiple choice questions and 5 multiple choice questions which included a section for additional remarks. The questionnaire was meant to obtain information regarding the following items:

1. The recorded variables: more/less/others desired (4 questions)
2. The subdivision in columns (2 questions)
3. The expansion of the layout with additional tables (1 question)
4. The number of variables to be plotted in graphs (2 questions)
5. The ranges for the graphs (2 questions)
6. The presentation of artifacts (1 question)
7. The event marking (1 question)
8. The use of colors (1 question)
9. The desirability of units (1 question)
10. The frequency of numerical recording of automatically sampled data (1 question)

To be assured of valid, useful answers and to eliminate possible confusion amongst the interviewees, strict rules were followed when formulating the questions. The rules were derived in a study into the efficient method of information extraction (van der Stap 1982). Some rules:

- Use alternating types of questions.
- Before formulating the question determine what the information is that has to be extracted by the question.
- Take the foreknowledge of the respondent into account.
- In a two-way question or a multiple choice question either all alternatives have to be explicitly given, or none at all.
- Keep the questions short.

The questionnaire was handed out to 30 staff anesthesiologists and residents familiar with thoracical procedures. It was accompanied by a sample anesthesia record and an introduction to explain the questionnaire and the design constraints underlying the automated record.

Results: Seventeen completed questionnaires (57%) were returned. One of the thirteen anesthesiologists who did not respond claimed not to have enough knowledge about DADS to complete the questionnaire. The remaining 12 gave no explanation for their lack of participation but possible reasons are:

1) not enough experience with DADS (though knowledge of DADS was not necessary),
2) not interested,
3) forgotten/lack of time,
4) bad questionnaire.

Of the returned questions, all were answered and the most relevant deductions with respect to the ten items mentioned above will be discussed:

1. - As soon as a cardiac output value is entered, DADS computes derived variables such as the cardiac index (CI = CO/Body Surface Area) and the systemic vascular resistance (SVR = (MAP-MCVP)/CO). It would be appreciated if these values were plotted in the CO column.
   - The graphical presentation of the diastolic pulmonary pressure (DPAP) was favored above the mean pulmonary pressure (MPAP) because the former is a better representation of the mean left atrial pressure. Currently, the only reason that the DPAP is not plotted is that it is not (yet) available at an output port of the front-end rack.
2. - To enhance the presentation of administered drugs it seems useful to divide the pharmaca column into a column for drugs administered in a bolus and drugs administered with an infusion pump.
   - A fluid-balance column for drip infusions, urine production and blood loss/transfusions should be placed at the left of the comment column.
   - The comment column is too wide.
3. - No comment
4. - Though not the majority, 7 respondents preferred a graph of the CO_2ex. Two others wanted more detailed information on the CO_2ex in case of problems, and one preferred the real-time capnogram.
5. - Nine respondents opted for a wider range for systemic blood pressures and heart rate. This enables the presentation of more deviating values but at the expense of the resolution of the majority of the graphs. One solution might be to plot all graphs on one scale along one vertical axis. This would increase the resolution for the arterial pressures and heart rate but decrease the resolution for MCVP and MPAP, to which there is probably no objection.
6. - Currently actions such as flushing, sampling and cardiac output measurements give rise to an artifact in the plotted signals. It seems desirable to mark the artifacts, for instance with an arrow at the corresponding point in the graph. Removal of the artifacts from the graphs might then be considered.
7. - We suggest marking an event in a separate column near the time axis of the graph, possibly with the serial number.
8. - The respondents were almost unanimously positive on the usefulness of colors in the record.
9. - The majority (11) of the respondents did not consider units to be necessary; however, for scientific reasons they will be added anyway.
10. - One interesting answer regarding the rate with which the numerical values are plotted was given; at the moment this is every 10 minutes and in the case of an event: it was suggested that it should be possible to choose this rate during the operation.

Conclusion: The principle of arranging the main part of the record in columns will remain unchanged, but there will be some changes within the columns. In particular the plotting of additional variables in graphs (CO_2ex and perhaps also temperatures) and the readjusted range for the blood pressures and heart rate will give the record a somewhat different appearance. Moreover, the presentation of artifacts and events will be reconsidered, units will be added to the headers, the comment column will be made narrower and plotting of SVR and CI values will be combined with the plotting of CO values. The tables below the record will remain.

7.4 Discussion

The first attempts at generating an automated record were made by American researchers toward the end of the 1970s (Newbower 1985 priv. comm.). Currently, with the introduction of automation in European ORs, automated records have been designed independently at at least five institutes (Hartung et al. 1983, Karliczek et al. 1985, van Kessel et al. 1986, Prakash et al. 1984, Trispel et al. 1985).

Though it will take some time before commercial applications are in common use, it is to be expected that there will be much interest in this new development. This is not surprising when we consider the time required for handwritten record keeping and the dubious quality of the result.

An important constraint for the expected time saving at the moment is that, as yet, many variables have to be entered into the system manually: this will change with progressive automation in the hospitals. Again, among the designs of automated records, differences in layout are manifest; these will only be eliminated if attempts to standardize are made. Whether this is necessary is questionable as the most important objectives of an automated record have already been realized, namely legibility, objectivity, and completeness.

8 Critical Incidents: A Postscript

8.1 Introduction

In this book the concept of critical incidents has been emphasized a number of times. The concept as such is rather new and was only recently introduced by Cooper et al. (1978), in the form of a study in which the "critical-incident technique" (Flanagan 1954) was applied to anesthesia management. Until that time, terms such as "mishaps" and "adverse occurrences" etc. had been used in studies which exclusively discussed anesthesia procedures with a fatal outcome.

Below I will label the different studies as either "critical-incident" or "mortality", but when both indications apply I will use the term "mishap". The reason why studies with respect to critical incidents are so important has been formulated as follows by Newbower et al. (1981b): "The present level of risk in anesthesia, while small, is not irreducible... Quite possibly, a more systematic approach to the analysis of errors and failures and to the design of corrective action could help to produce a better anesthesia result", and: "Preventing the problems related to human factors and equipment failures which lead to near-miss incidents is believed to reduce the probability of ultimate disaster."

In Chapter 4 critical incidents were mentioned both in relation to performance criteria and (re)design criteria for automated monitoring systems. The use of critical incidents as a criterion to measure the performance of a system was not considered to be feasible.

However, a systematic analysis of circumstances and patient signals in the operating room was performed in this book in order to select those aspects where the use of automation may ultimately lead to a decrease in critical incidents. In the scope of redesign a number of suggestions for improvement of information presentation in the OR by means of automation were given in Chapter 2. Some of these improvements may prevent smaller adverse occurrences which may lead to a critical incident. In Chapter 5 it was shown that specific signal behavior precedes certain clinically significant events, and an investigation into the use of signal correlations to warn for some critical incidents was recommended.

Based on the suggestions from Chapter 2, Chapter 6 discussed the (re)design of an integrated workstation. It represents our view on the direction in which the layout of operating rooms should go in order to minimize errors associated with both scattered information presentation and instrument control.

With the objective of reaching a reduction in peroperative mortality and morbidity, a direct study of critical incidents might well lead to useful recommendations with respect to automation in the operating room and could perhaps yield clues regarding the requirements for alarm algorithms.

For example, a disconnection of the tracheal tube is a frequently occurring incident; it can be prevented by a special mechanical construction (Pogulanik 1980), but also by providing an alarm triggered by the signal behavior resulting from the disconnection (McEwen and Jenkins 1983).

In this chapter I will mention some of the most important publications on the subject of mishaps. Furthermore, I will list the results from 6 recent survey studies in order to obtain an indication of the mishap incidence and thereby of those aspects which most urgently require the application of automation (Meijler et al. 1982). A few illustrative suggestions will be given, although I will do this with some reservations: publications on the subject of mishaps are innumerable and the diversity of the performed investigations is such that comparing and using their results is a precarious enterprise. An adequate description of this literature and its use for automation in anesthesia merits a book of its own, and I will restrict myself to a tentative reconnaissance.

8.2 Critical Incidents as a Means

Several authors give outstanding reviews of the literature regarding mishaps in anesthesia (Phillips and Capizzi 1974, Keats 1979, Davies and Strunin 1984, Pierce 1984). In the history of anesthesia the first reported mishap occurred in 1848, well over a year after the first administration of an anesthetic. Apart from a remarkable mortality study by Snow published in 1858, all subsequent studies were primarily "case reports, compilations of case reports, or collections of compilations" (Phillips and Capizzi 1974). The first systematic survey was published by Beecher and Todd in 1954: they investigated 599,500 surgical procedures and divided the 384 cases of anesthesia-associated mortality into different categories according to their cause. An enormous wave of publications followed. In the period between 1980 and 1985 alone, more than 50 articles were published. Roughly, they can be divided in three groups: those describing specific equipment problems such as Cooper and Newbower (1975) and Rendell-Baker (1982) on anesthesia machines, case studies (Gordh and Mostert 1978), and survey studies of mishaps. It is generally considered useful to compare results of the surveys to obtain improvements in anesthesia. However, one main problem is caused by the differences in the study methodology followed. This discussion about the uniformity of the collected data was initiated by Collins (1960): "The lack of uniformity in compilation of operating room statistics makes it difficult to appraise complications and death occurring in patients who undergo anesthetic and surgical procedures."

In the Netherlands, Smalhout (1972) listed the results from seven mortality studies and concluded: "Although there are large differences between the outcomes, there are some causes of mortality which reoccur in every study". According to him many mishaps could have been prevented by better organization, more knowledge about the situation, improved technical equipment and more careful management.

Phillips and Capizzi (1974) mention some of the differences in data collection, such as the period over which the data were collected, the patient populations, and the applied classifications. The major problem in obtaining comparable results is the lack of uniformity in classifications. In an ECRI technology assessment (1985) it is stated that: "no two studies have used identical classification systems to analyze the factors underlying anesthesia deaths".

The problem of classification can be illustrated as follows: an incident can originate at many different places in the total setting of men and equipment in the operating theatre. After its origination the incident evolves. This means that different people can easily have different interpretations and indicate different instants and/or different places for the origination of the incident.

An example: due to haste, a gastric tube has been placed incorrectly, resulting in aspiration of gastric contents followed by respiratory failure. Some investigators will give as cause the misplaced gastric tube; others, the aspiration; and again others will classify this mishap as inappropriate airway maintenance. In fact, all this information is essential for describing the mishap. When we combine the suggestions of the various authors for a complete classification, haste should be listed as the reason or associated factor, the misplaced gastric tube and (thus) inappropriate airway maintenance as cause, the aspiration is the direct consequence and respiratory failure the subsequent consequence.

Until now the classifications of causes, associated factors and consequences have often been confused which has resulted in very different outcomes. This complexity in pinpointing the causes was also confirmed by a study performed in New South Wales (1970), which says that an average of 4.3 mistakes preceded patient death.

Irrespective of all the problems originating in the various methods of data collection which were applied in the surveys, we decided to compare the outcomes of some of them. To this end, six surveys were selected in which causes, associated factors and consequences were not confused, or not to any great extent. These six surveys are given in Table 8.1. However, the classifications of causes in these studies were still different. Thus, to enable a global comparison between the data, the causes as determined in these studies were converted to a generalized classification in which all could be fitted. Table 8.2 presents an example: on the left, the classification as used by Craig and Wilson (1981) and on the right, our generalized classification, to which we converted the causes.

Table 8.1 Specifications of six studies on mishaps during anesthesia

Period of data collection	65-69	67-76	70-75	75	?	75-84?
Number of mishaps on which data are based	47	53	348	67	81	809
Number of concerning surgical procedures	34145	240483	?	338934	8312	?
	m*	m	m	m	c.i.	c.i.
	Marx et al. '73	Harrison '78	Utting et al. '79	Hovi-Viander '80	Craig and Wilson '81	Cooper et al. '84

* The m stands for mortality study and ci for critical-incident study.

Table 8.2 An example of the conversion of results from a mishap study (Craig and Wilson 1981) to a generalized classification.

Craig and Wilson	Meijler
Transmission of anesthetic gases and vapors: disconnections	Dis- or wrong connection in breathing system
Tracheal tube connector problem	
Tracheal tube problem: intubation cuff/pilot tube	Problems with in- and extubation
Transmission of anesthetic gases and vapors: obstruction	Inappropriate airway maintenance
Gas supply problems	Incorrect gasflow
Leaks in transmission of anesthetic gases	
Valve problems	
Halothane/trilene left on from previous case	Drug administration
Inaccurate calibration vaporizer	
Drug swap	
Drug omission	
Overdose/unnecessary drug	
*	Inadequate fluid replacement
IV-route problem: air in drip line	IV-apparatus
IV in wrong arm	
*	Monitoring problems
Miscellaneous	Others

* Mishaps from other surveys fall into this category of the generalized classification, but this is not the case with mishaps classified by Craig and Wilson.

It is a matter of course that, to enable this conversion, our classification had to be less specific (more generalized). The conversion tables for the remaining studies are given in Manteleers (1985). The resulting mishap incidences of the six studies with respect to the generalized classification are given in Table 8.3. The first six columns present the incidence of the mishaps for each study in percentages. Because all studies now have a common classification, the incidences can be compared.

The next two columns give the weighted means of, respectively, the mortality and the critical incident studies. The mean of both the mortality and the critical incident studies is given in the last column. The number of mishaps on which the studies are based determines the weighting of the study results in the computation of the mean. Although there is a considerable variation between the incidences (as expected), the mishaps with the highest incidence can be seen clearly. Most mishaps occur in relation to:

- incorrect gasflow (22.6%)
- drug administration (16.6%)
- problems with in and extubation (11.7%)

Inappropriate airway maintenance and dis- or wrong connection also make a considerable contribution, with more than 7% each.

As a possible reason for the differences between critical-incident and mortality results we want to mention a reason which stands apart from the differences in

Table 8.3 The incidence of mishaps in percentages according to our classification as based upon six surveys

Author / Category	Marx et al. '73	Harrison '78	Utting et al. '79	Hovi-Viander '80	Craig and Wilson '81	Cooper et al. '84	Weighted mean mort.	Weighted mean c.i.	Weighted mean mort. and c.i.
1: Dis- or wrong connection.	–	–	3.2	1.5	13.5	9.8	2.4	10.1	7.3
2: Problems with in- and extubation.	38.4	17.0	14.4	11.5	20.9	7.7	16.5	8.9	11.7
3: Inappr. airway maintenance.	13.8	22.7	7.4	11.5	1.2	6.8	10.1	6.3	7.7
4: Incorrect gasflow.	13.8	1.9	8.4	11.5	27.1	31.1	8.6	30.7	22.6
5: Drug administration.	14.9	26.4	16.7	1.5	18.6	17.1	15.6	17.2	16.6
6: Inadequate fluid replacement.	6.4	7.6	1.7	26.9	–	3.8	6.0	3.5	4.4
7: IV apparatus.	–	1.9	–	–	2.4	6.8	0.2	6.4	4.1
8: Monitoring problems.	–	–	–	–	–	7.1	0	6.5	4.1
9: Others.	12.7	22.7	48.1	35.8	16.0	9.8	40.6	10.4	21.5
	mortality				c.i.				

study methodology as discussed above. This concerns the different sensitivity of critical-incident and mortality studies for a fatal outcome. Some mishaps may occur often and be recorded as a critical incident but they do not always result in a fatal outcome. For instance, a critical incident with the gas flow occurs very frequently (30.7%), although in the majority of the cases it does not lead to a fatal outcome (8.6%).

We mentioned before that causes, associated factors and consequences are all essential to describe a mishap. Several authors have investigated which factors are those most frequently associated with the observed incidents (Cooper et al. 1984, Craig and Wilson 1981, Lunn and Mushin 1982):

- lack of experience
- inadequate familiarity with the equipment
- haste
- omission of routine inspections
- fatigue
- lack of communication with colleagues

Suggestions: Above we presented the main causes and associated factors which are related to mishaps. With respect to further research on the application of automation, we think that further research on the mishaps in categories 1.(dis- or wrong connection), 4.(incorrect gasflow) and 5.(drug administration) should be instigated.

Many of the mishaps in categories 1. and 4. may be prevented by the application of existing monitoring devices such as oxygen analyzers, CO_2 analyzers and by ventilation and disconnect alarms (Spooner and Kirby 1984, Duberman and Bendixen 1984). The former also recommend the use of better equipment checks (see below).

Our opinion is that, as a first step an automated system could take care of the central presentation of alarms generated by these devices. This could be easily implemented in DADS.

The positioning of additional sensors at some other critical places in the routes of the gases to the patient must also be considered, for instance to prevent N_2O instead of O_2 supply (Footerman 1983). Central alarming facilities can again be provided for by the computer.

The prevention of errors in drug administration (category 5) (Warner et al. 1985, Harrison and Ludwig 1983) and fluid replacement (category 6) is, in our opinion, a tremendous challenge for physicians and engineers alike. An extension to future monitoring systems is needed, which could take the form of a software package which performs checks on the administered drugs and fluids, and alarms when necessary. For this to function, the system will need information about demographic data, patient history, allergies, pharmacokinetics and type of operation. The easy entry of these data into a computer requires further steps in the automation of hospitals. On that subject, suggestions have already been given in Section 2.5 (networking) and 6.2.3 (bar-code labelling). In Section 3.8 we mentioned the planned medical data display facility which was developed for DADS. This display will present all the interventions, including the administered drugs and fluids with the corresponding cumulative doses. If limits were known to the system, a message could be generated when these were exceeded. With respect to the associated factors, we think that the improvements as suggested in Chapter 2 may deal with the lack of communication. To prevent the omission of routine inspections we refer to the checklist as published by Spooner and Kirby (1984). Such a list could easily be generated by an automated system in the operating room. As far as necessary the system can ensure the acknowledgement by the anesthesiologists or the technicians of the points on the list. Further strategies into the prevention of associated factors which do not belong to the scope of this book are given by Cooper et al. (1984).

8.3 Discussion

Above, we were able to give a number of recommendations for future automated patient-monitoring systems. Because of the generalized classification which had to be applied to enable comparison of the outcomes, some details from the surveys were lost and recommendations could only be given in general terms. Much effort has yet to be spent on research before implementation of the suggestions can be effected. Some of these ideas, or parts of them, are also recognized by the industry. For example, programs are being developed for the computation and updating of drug administration and fluid balance records.

The classification problem was extensively discussed in a symposium in Boston on preventable mortality and morbidity. Several suggestions for classifications have been given (Keats and Siker 1985): "For example, the mechanism (process) of a harmful outcome was described by one contributor as a cascade initiated by an occurrence, followed by a potentially harmful outcome, a complication and a final outcome. Intervention may halt the cascade at any point, and these interventions require classification. Another participant defined undesirable outcomes in therapy, diagnostic costs, and length of stay in terms of deviations from expectations of the patient and the physician. Other approaches were based on classification by organ affected, by anesthesia management area (airway, circulation, drugs) or simply a list of all adverse anesthesia occurrences". But, according to Keats (1979), even when the errors could be correctly identified "all published estimates of their incidence are unacceptable" because there are mishaps which are not preventable and thus should not be included in the results. In addition, Cooper et al. (1978) make a distinction between equipment failure and human errors.

In our opinion, many of the above-mentioned problems incurred during the classification of mishaps can be avoided if causes, reasons, or associated factors and consequences are clearly discriminated and each has its own classification.

For the causes, we believe that a classification in which both topological and chronological aspects are interwoven might be useful. For instance, with respect to drug administration the classification could be:

- drug supplies
- drug storage in OR
- drug preparation (peroperatively)
- drug administration

We suggest, partly based on Cooper et al. (1979), that the main classification of associated factors could be:

- whether the incident is workplace-induced, that is, caused by the spatial arrangement of the equipment
- design-induced, that is, resulting from equipment failure or characteristics enhancing the probability of error
- operator-induced, caused by inadequacies of individuals
- organization-induced, caused by shortcomings in the hospital, or OR organization.
- procedure-induced, long surgical procedure etc.

Finally: for the future we again recommend the utilization of the computer as a centralized collecting system. It should be applied not exclusively for monitoring and processing of patient signals (as already effected by DADS), but should also register and process information on administered drugs and fluids. Furthermore, the control, readout, and checking of all anesthesia and monitoring devices should take place by means of this system. It must be realized that human errors can never be completely avoided; an important contribution of automation in anesthesia is to help alleviate unwanted or dangerous consequences of such errors.

Summary

This book contains a systematic treatment of computers in patient monitoring. The basis for this approach forms the development, clinical evaluation and ergonomic revision of a Data Acquisition and Display System (DADS) for patient monitoring during anesthesia. DADS was developed with the aim of improving deficiencies in the organization of information presentation and the low standard of information processing in the operating rooms (Chapter 3).

Particularly during cardioanesthesia, on which this book focuses, the number of patient variables to be monitored may amount to up to 30, and their presentation is various and scattered. Nevertheless the anesthesiologist is expected to make the correct decisions swiftly and to act accordingly. In this book the work situation of the anesthesiologist in the operating room was systematically described (Chapter 2), whereby it became clear that efficient task performance is almost impossible. A number of recommendations for improvement by means of automation could be given (Section 2.5).

Some examples:

- The automated acquisition, processing and centralized display of measurement data should not exclusively concern the anesthesia equipment, but also, for instance, the cardiopulmonary bypass apparatus. Transfer of information between such devices should be possible as well. This aspect will not be elaborated in this book.
- The criterion of centralized and comprehensive presentation of information should also be met by the layout of the equipment controls. This implies that further integration and adjustment of equipment is required. To give expression to our recommendations on this point, a design of a new "maxi-DADS" was realized in collaboration with a commercial partner. The steps leading to the design of the "maxi-DADS" are comparable with those for the cockpit of an aircraft (Chapter 6). In that same chapter ergonomic guidelines for information presentation (use of color, legibility) and operation of such a workstation are given.
- It was found that the need existed for a reduction of the workload by the automatic generation of an anesthesia record. In addition, such a record promised to be much more objective and legible than the handwritten record. Therefore an automated record was implemented which, according to a questionnaire submitted to the users, clearly lived up to the expectations.

The deficiencies as described in Chapter 2 and the revisions of DADS induced by them, all form part of a generally applicable evaluation method which we developed and applied to DADS (Chapter4). This method gives a strategy which prescribes in the first place knowledge-acquisition on the subjects of task analysis, ergonomics and critical incidents. Armed with this knowledge, we composed the criteria both for redesign of the system and for testing its (clinical) performance.

Two important facilities of DADS have been subjected to clinical testing (Chapter5):

1. An alarm algorithm that warns of fast changes has been implemented in DADS. The generated warnings were related to the actions of the anesthesiologists in order to determine the usefulness of the warnings. It was shown that useful warnings can be expected mainly for unexpected problems with the equipment or catheters, at the occurrence of stress-arousing interventions, and after the administration of (vasoactive) drugs. We demonstrated that it must be possible, because of their deviating signal pattern, to suppress some of the false warnings which are triggered by artifacts. We also postulate that, by making sure that the system is (automatically) provided with the time and character of medical interventions, the percentage of useful warnings can be increased. In spite of these measures, we expect that for the time being the number of useful warnings will remain between 10% and 20%. This is not surprising when we take into account that the study revealed only about two fast signal changes per hour which are sufficiently clinically significant to cause a warning. We estimated that in addition, some 10 slow, clinically significant changes per procedure occur. The continuous trend presentation in DADS (graphical display) contributed to the detection of these unwanted slow changes.

2. In a second test we investigated whether the system display of DADS that is based on the principle of the 'artificial horizon' (bar display) has an influence on the behavior of the hemodynamic signals as measured at the patient. Although no significant conclusions could be drawn from the small population investigated, the expectation was confirmed that controllability of anesthesia depends only to a minor degree on the monitoring equipment and to a much greater extent on the type of patient, his preoperative status, and the attending anesthesiologist. However, we noticed that an experienced anesthesiologist tended to have a lower error of control when using DADS. In addition a better picture of the way in which variables are controlled was obtained. Not all signals receive the same attention during control. In general, most effort was put into the control of the systemic arterial pressures. The mean pulmonary pressure shows, especially at induction, apparently poorly controllable peaks. The mean central venous pressure mainly shows smaller changes and reacts slowly. In this signal the trends seem to be most important.

Further improvements in alarm algorithms can be achieved by using correlations between signals. At the moment, the knowledge gained from the present study is being applied in an expert system which will be developed in subsequent research within the division, with the goal of raising alarm algorithms to a more intelligent level.

Finally, we wish to stress the important recommendation that aspects to which automation might be most effectively applied are those where the most critical incidents occur. Critical incidents are defined as those mishaps which, if not recognized and obviated in time, could be detrimental to the patient. Aspects to which automation should be initially applied are, among other things drug administration, incorrect gasflows, and disconnections in the breathing circuit.

On the whole, the investigations described were successful in leading to an objective charting of anesthesis management and the corresponding signal behavior. This proved to be very useful in achieving improvements in monitoring.

APPENDIX 1

The Anesthesia Activity Chart

SURGEON

Actions	Monitoring	Drugs
Scrub hands		
Introduction of urinary catheter		

PUMP-TECHNICIAN

	4 Actions	5 Monitoring	6 Drugs
1			
2			
3			
4			
5			
6			
7			
8			
9			
10			
11			
12			
13			
14			
15			
16			
17			
18			
19			
20	Check OR equipment		
21			
22	Prepare transducers		
23	and catheters		
24			
25	ECG leads on recorder		
26			
27			
28			
29			
30			
31			
32			
33			
34	Prepare Cardio-Pulmonary		
35	Bypass Apparatus		
36			
37			
38			
39			
40			
41			
42			
43			
44			
45			
46			
47			
48			
49			
50			
51			
52			
53			
54			
55			
56			
57			
58			
59			
60			
61			
62			
63			
64			
65			
66			
67			
68			
69			
70			
71			
72			
73			
74			
75	Scrub patient		
76			
77			
78			
79			

7	8	9
TIME	ANESTHESIOLOGIST	
	Actions	Monitoring
Previous day	Check patient chart	
	Preoperative visit	Allens test for patency radial arteries
		Check temperature
		Check patency nasal airway
		Coronary angiograms
		Catheterization data
		Labresults: Hb-> oxygen saturation Potassium-> prevention of arrhythmias
		Coagulation
Preceding procedure		
	Check OR equipment	
Patient in OR		
	Attach ECG electrodes including V5 lead	Check signal quality, initial value HR
	Adjust transducers and calibrate	ischemia
	Introduce two peripheral IV cannulae	
	Introduce one arterial catheter	Check signal quality, initial pattern PART wavefor
	Apply one long central catheter (slow drug administration)	
	Bloodsample	
	Apply cuff for noninvasive bloodpressure measurements	Additional noninvasive measurement
	Introduce Jugular or Swan-Ganz catheter (depending on LV function)	Check signal quality initial value of MCVP or RA pressure
	In case of Swan-Ganz perform Cardiac Output (CO) measurement	
	Induction of anesthesia	PART,HR,ECG reaction patient (circulation) on induction
		DPAP ischemia
	Laryngoscopy	PART,HR
	Intubation (first strong stress arousing intervention)	Listen to air entry L,R lungs DPAP
	Start ventilation	Check humidifier
		MCVP
	Connect CO2 analyzer	
	Introduce gastric-tube	Listening, suctioning of gastric contents
	Apply thermistor probes peripheral toe, thumb central nasopharynx	
	Sometimes Jugular or Swan-Ganz catheter catheter after induction	RA,PAP,DPAP
	Screen	
	Bloodsamples-> electrolytes, bloodgases	
	ACT	
	Protect patients eyes	

	10	11	12
			ANESTHETIC NURSE
	Motivation	Drugs	
1			
2			
3			
4			
5			
6			
7			
8			
9		Evening-medication	
10			
11		Premedication	
12			
13			
14			
15			
16			
17			
18			
19			
20			
21			
22			Check equipment
23			
24			
25			
26			
27			
28			
29			Apply ECG electrodes
30			
31			
32			
33			
34		Dripp infusions	Insert 2 peripheral IV'
35			
36			Insert 1 arterial cathe
37			
38		Dopamine (once before induction)	Insert 1 long intravenc
39			catheter
40			Prepare drugs
41			
42			
43			
44			
45			
46			
47	Watch for bradycardia	100% O2 spontaneous respiration	
48		Fentanyl	
49		O2+N2O manual ventilation	
50		Anesthetica+Muscle relaxants	
51			
52		Antibiotic	
53	Stress?	Lidocaine spray of	
54		larynx and trachea	
55	Correct placement of tube		
56	If elevated, LV function		
57	inadequate. Some NTG may		
58	be administered		
59	Filling		
60			
61			
62		Spray Lidocaine	
63			
64			
65			
66			
67			
68			
69			
70			
71			
72			
73			
74			
75			(Scrub)
76			
77			
78			
79			

1	2	3
SURGEON		
Actions	Monitoring	Drugs
Draping patient		
Incision leg		
Incision skin thorax	ECG,HR,PART,CVP,PAP	
Sternotomy	Temp stop Ventilation	
Sternal spread		
Cautery haemostasis		
Dissection of mediastinum		
Opening pericardium	Blood color	
		Heparin in Right Atrium
Cannulation aorta		
Cannulation of Vena Cava		
Inferior and Superior		
Cannula in Left Ventricle		
Cannula cardioplegic solution		
		Surface cooling heart
Identification and inspection	Flow and Volume in lungs	
of coronary arteries	Electrical activity	
	of the heart	
Aortic cross clamp		
Distal anastomosis		
Operation		Fluid suctioning
Aortic clamp off		
Defibrillation (if required)	ECG, HR	
Introduction catheter	Intracardiac pressures	
in Left Atrium		
(if no Swan Ganz)		
Anastomose proximal grafts		
Epicardial pacemaker		
(if required)		
Surgical venting	Prevent cerebral air-embolism	
Decannulation of:		
LV,		
VCI, VCS		
Aorta		
Closing Pericardium		
Sternum		
Subcutaneous tissues		
Skin		

PUMP-TECHNICIAN

	4 Actions	5 Monitoring	6 Drugs
82	Draping patient		
100			Heparin,Mannitol,antibiotics
101			in pump
107			Muscle relaxants
108	Start bypass -> cooling	Flow, Shim, line pressure	and vasoactive drugs just
109		Bubbles, Temperatures	before bypass
110	Sampling for bloodgas	Cardiotomy	
111	every 15 to 30 minutes		
112	Sample for Activated		
113	Clotting Time		
114	once every ten minutes		Nitroprusside
115	Cardioplegic solution		
116	once every 30 minutes		
117	Start monitoring Capno		
122	Warming	ECG, HR	
129	Weaning (decrease pumpflow)		
137	Bring cardiac filling		
138	to required level		
140	Stop bypass		
148	Clearing away of Bypass		
149	Apparatus		
157	Prepare patient for bed		

	7	8	9
	TIME	ANESTHESIOLOGIST	
		Actions	Monitoring
80		Measure CO (if SG)(vent stop)	Computation of LVSWI,SVR,SI
81			
82			
83			
84			
85			
86			
87			
88			
89			
90			Hemodynamic parameters
91			Difference between
92		Vent. stop->disconnect	peripheral and central
93		Measure CO	temperatures
94			
95			
96			
97			Pupil size
98			Urine output
99			
100			
101			
102			
103		Clear cart	
104			
105		ACT (every 10 min)	
106			
107			
108			Skin color patient
109		Adjust tidal volume-> 50%	MCVP,MPAP
110			
111			
112			
113			
114		Vent.stop. 5cmH2O PEEP	
115			
116		Clear cart,	HR,PART
117		perform delayed tasks	
118			
119			
120			
121		Start ventilation-> 50%	Urine output
122			ECG,HR
123			
124			
125			
126			
127			
128			Perspiration
129		ACT	
130			
131			
132			
133			
134			
135			
136			
137			
138		Ventilation 100%	
139			
140		CO measurement	
141		Sampling	
142		Bloodtransfusions	
143			
144			
145			
146			
147			
148			HR,PART
149			
150			
151			
152			
153			
154			
155			
156		Prepare patient for bed	
157	Subsequent		
158	to procedure	Patient to ICU	

	10	11	12
			ANESTHETIC NURSE
	Motivation	Drugs	
80			(Place suction reserv
81			
82			(Draping)
83			
84			
85			
86			
87			
88			
89		Anticipating	
90		anesthetics and vasoactive	
91		drugs	
92			
93	For estimating SVR if no SG		
94			
95			
96			
97			
98			
99		Heparin	
100		Calcium solution	
101		for filling and contraction	
102			Clear cart
103			
104			
105			
106			
107			
108	Because start bypass		
109			
110			
111			
112			
113		Stop N2O administration	
114			
115			Prepare drugs
116			(protamine,dopamine e
117			
118			
119			
120			
121			
122			
123			
124			
125			
126			
127			
128	Sympathetic activity		
129			
130			
131			
132			
133			
134			
135			
136			
137			
138	In anticipation of Protamine	Calcium (frequently)	
139	Possible low PART caused by		
140	filling or dilation	Protamine reversal	
141	To restore filling,Hb,Ht		
142		Dopamine if necessary	
143		for stimulating contractility	
144	For removing excess of CPB fluid	Diuretics	
145	if low urine output	combined with Potassium	
146	or high filling pressure		
147		Fentanyl if required	
148			
149			
150			
151			
152			
153			
154			
155			Prepare patient for b
156			
157			
158			

Appendix 2

A Survey of Events During Coronary Bypass Surgery

The events are given in alphabetical order. The events marked with an asterisk give rise to an artifact and can be marked by the operator of DADS by means of the artifact button.

Activated Clotting Time (ACT), start determination
Activated Clotting Time, readout value
Blood transfusion
Bypass start
Bypass stop
Calibration *
Cannulation aorta
Cannulation Left Ventricle
Cannulation Inferior Vena Cava
Cannulation Superior Vena Cava
Capno-line pinched
Cardiac Output (CO) determination *
Cardioplegia
Change flow
Change perfusor setting
Change ventilator setting
Clamping aorta
Clamp from aorta
Decannulation aorta
Decannulation Left Ventricle
Decannulation Inferior Vena Cava
Decannulation Superior Vena Cava
Defibrillation
Disconnect ventilator
Draping
Drug administration
ECG electrode disconnected
Fibrillation
Fluid infusion (intravenous)
Flushing *
Incision
Induction
Intubation
Laryngoscopy
Manipulation heart
Pacemaker on
Pacemaker off
Pericardium open
Pericardium closed
Sampling arterial line *

Sampling venous line *
Scrub
Side-clamp aorta
Side-clamp from aorta
Sternotomy
Sternal spread
Sternal spread maximal
Sternal closing start
Sternal closed
Stomach-tube
Pulmonary arterial catheter manipulation *
Table head up
Table head down
Transducer plateau up *
Transducer plateau down *
Urinary catheter
Urinary production
Wedge

Appendix 3

The Disturbance Detection Algorithm: Backgrounds

Every second, the variables derived from the measurements at the patient (to be called data points or observations) are subjected to a check to determine whether they exceed their static alarm limits. These limits have been set by the user of the system and correspond to limits as presented on one of the displays of DADS. When a limit is exceeded the status too high (7) or too low (6) is attached to the variable and its presentation on the displays is enhanced.

If the variable is within the static limits it is checked for dynamic disturbances. This part of the algorithm was developed by Gieles (1978), Jorritsma et al. (1979) and Blom et al. (1981).

Gieles collected a set of signals from patients during gynaecological procedures. He found that within a period of two minutes, no significant trends appeared in these signals and the amplitude followed approximately a normal $N(\mu, \sigma^2)$ distribution. The running average $\bar{x}_k$ is an estimation of the mean of the distribution with

$$\bar{x}_{k+1} = \bar{x}_k + (x_{k+1} - \bar{x}_k)/t_x$$

The filterconstant t_x is set at 128 sec. (2^7). The mean deviation d_k is an estimation of the standard deviation (or more accurately $d_k \simeq 3/4\sigma$) with

$$d_{k+1} = d_k + (|x_{k+1} - \bar{x}_k| - d_k)/t_d$$

where filter constant t_d equals 1024 sec (2^{10}). The value for t_x was chosen to allow the assumption of normality and to ensure a good tracking of the signal corresponding to an accurate average, which, in turn, is essential for reliable values of d_k.

However, such a small filter constant should not be chosen for the mean deviation. The mean deviation would then follow the disturbances in the signal, instead of detecting them. In Fig. A.3.1 the flowchart of the algorithm is given.

The null hypothesis for the detection test is that the data points are taken from a normal probability distribution with parameter values estimated as indicated (above). It is rejected as soon as a sample x_{k+1} satisfies

$$|x_{k+1} - \bar{x}_k| > 4d_k$$

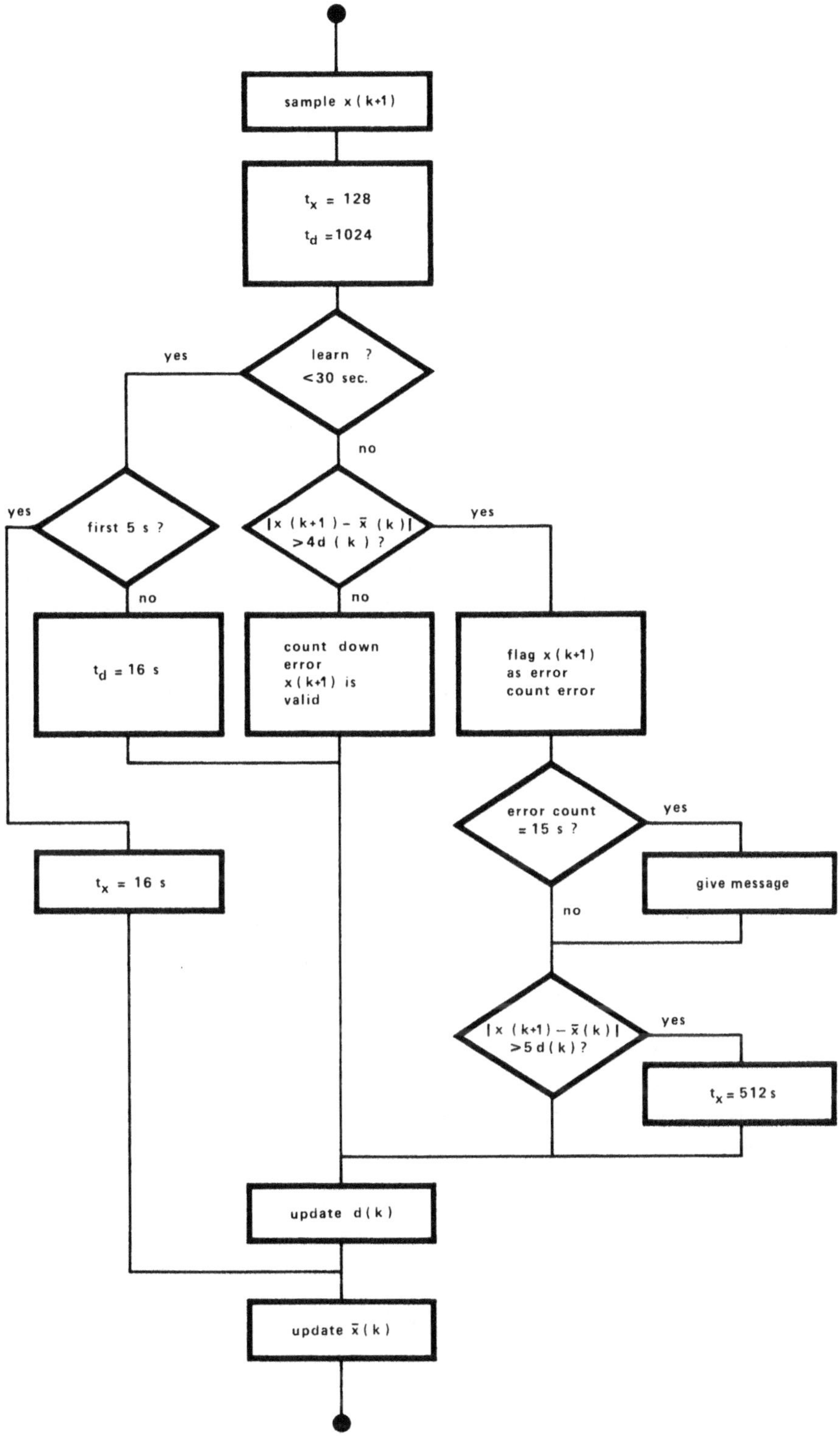

Fig. A.3.1 Flowchart of the disturbance detection algorithm.

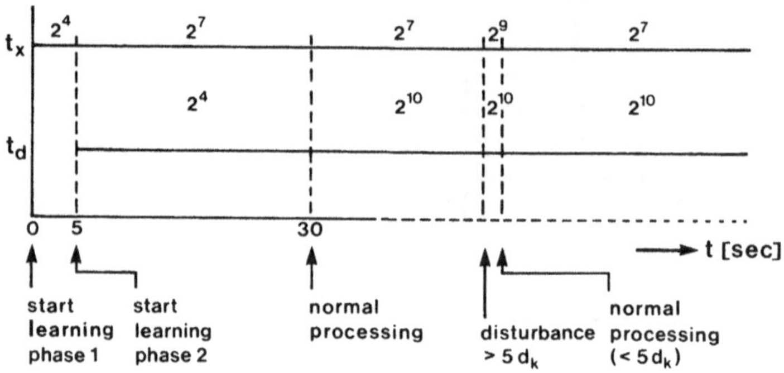

Fig. A.3.2 The values of the time constants t_x and t_k in the different conditions of the disturbance detection algorithm.

This is the same as saying that x_{k+1} is exceeding the confidence interval ranging from $-4d_k \rightarrow +4d_k$. Except for a probability of 2.8% one can then be sure to have detected a disturbance, assuming the assumptions of the signal model hold. When a data point exceeds a limit of $5\,d_k$ it notably widens the confidence interval and therewith reduces the chance for detection of the next disturbance. On the other hand it can be stated that except for a probability of .02%, it belongs to a disturbance. No big mistake is made in computing $\bar{x}_{k+1}$ if such a data point is weighted much less. Therefore, the filter constant t_x is increased to 512 sec. (2^9).

With each outlying data point a "disturbance counter" is incremented, up to a maximum of 15. This counter is decremented with each datapoint found within the confidence bands, down to zero. As soon as this counter is at 15, a message regarding the disturbance is generated.

Such a message reads for instance: "CO_2ex disturbed, above limit"

In two initial learning phases after a signal has been switched on, smaller time constants will result in accurate starting values for $\bar{x}_k$ and d_k within 30 sec. After this learning period normal processing begins with the original time constants (Fig. A.3.2).

The described algorithm detects strong, statistically significant disturbances. However it is intended to warn for situations which are also clinically significant. In Chapter 5 the outcome of the algorithm is compared with clinically significant situations.

Appendix 4

Artifact Suppression

As mentioned in Section 5.3.2, the operator of DADS marked occurring artifacts by means of a special key. The program for off-line computation of the surface areas was extended with a special subroutine for identifying those points around such a mark which belong to the artifact. If these are determined they can be excluded from the computation of the surface areas. To be able to suppress the artifacts it was necessary to determine whether the artifacts were composed of recurrent patterns. To this end we made a small inventory of the occurring artifacts for two of the studies.

The following points were recorded:

- begin time of artifact
- time of detection (marking) by the operator
- end time of artifact
- number of maxima respectively minima
- difference between the first and the last two successive samples
- minimal difference between two successive samples
- cause
- highest and lowest value
- number of samples
- number of samples with DADS state 4,5,6 or 7
- form of the artifact

From the inventory we concluded that, most artifacts have a duration of about one minute, however some last as long as three minutes. Artifacts may have only one extreme, however two maxima and one minimum are no exeption. Artifacts with more then one extreme often have a crossing with the (DADS) confidence interval (width for artifact detection at 3 times the mean deviation of the signal around the running average). However, this crossing consists mostly of one sample. Two successive samples within the confidence interval generally mark the end of the artifact. The start of an artifact, i.e. the samples preceding the artifact marking, are only part of the artifact if, from artifact mark looking backwards, they lie consistently outside the confidence interval. The number of samples preceding the artifact mark does not generally exceed four (or one minute).

Based on these conclusions we designed an artifact suppression algorithm. To this end four samples preceding an artifact mark and eight samples following the artifact mark have to be tested against criteria to determine whether they belong to the artifact. To keep up with this administration we mark the 5 most recent samples with a pointer: four samples corresponding to the accepted maximum length of one minute before the artifact mark; one pointer for the most recent sample. With each new sample the pointers are shifted one place. By means of these pointers we are able to delay the whole off-line data processing with four samples. This must be done, since upon detection of an artifact mark the four preceding samples must first be checked before further surface computation can take place. Thus, previous to the computation of the surface areas the program REPORT scans the data on occurrence of the artifact mark and marks the data points which are part of it.

In pseudofortran:

```
For I = 1,4 do
        if XT(pntr(5-i)) > AVT + 3*DEVT
          Pflag(pntr(5-i)) = .false.
```

Thus at the moment of identification of the last sample (pntr5) processing does not yet take place on this sample but on the sample detected one minute previously (pntr1) and then only when that sample is accompanied by a flag which indicates whether processing is allowed (pflag(pntr1) = .true.).

Also eight samples following the artifact are checked against the same criterion:

```
For     PACNTR = 8 down till 0
If      XT(pntr(5)) > AVT + 3*DEVT
Then    Pflag(pntr(5)) = .false.
```

the first sample for which holds that

XT(pntr(5)) < AVT + 3*DEVT still gets the Pflag = .false. mark. This enables the detection of an artifact with two extremes. As soon as two adjacent samples both lie within the confidence limit, or only one which, however, is the last data point in the series of eight, these are marked with Pflag(pntr(5)) and Pflag(pntr(4)) = .true.. The artifact is considered to be over.

Remark 1: In the case of two subsequent artifacts, the data points marked as unfit for surface computation by the first artifact are blocked for remarking by the next artifact. Also data points which were marked as not belonging to the first artifact as yet can be marked as unfit by the next.

Remark 2: Data points which are marked as unfit for surface area computation are also considered as unfit for updating of running average and mean deviation. In consequence it may happen that, when the signal behavior lies on a somewhat different level following an artifact, it can last a long time before AVT and DEVT return to realistic values. This of course influences the detection of artifacts over these periods.

Remark 3: Sometimes it may occur that the operator misses an artifact. To prevent these artifacts from distorting the controllability values, the algorithm for artifact suppression is also initiated when one of the variables exceeds a certain limit. These limits were set at 200 mmHg for PART, 40 mmHg for MPAP and 20 mmHg for MCVP. No separate limit was set for the HR because of its close relationship with the artifacts in PART.

References

Alcover IA, Henning RJ, Jackson DL (1984). A computer-assisted monitoring system for arrhythmia detection in a medical intensive care unit. Crit Care Med 12: 888-891

Arbeidsinspectie (1979). Het werken met beeldschermen. Concept voorlichtingsblad. Uitgave Directoraat-Generaal v.d. Arbeid v.h. Ministerie van Sociale Zaken, Postbox 69, Voorburg.

ASA newsletter (1985). Guidelines for patient care in anesthesiology. (Amended by House of Delegates on October 16) 49 no 12: 8

Baetz WR, Schneider AJL, Apple H, Fadel J, Katona P (1979). The anesthesia keyboard system. In: Gravenstein JS, Newbower RS, Ream AK, Smith NT, Barden J eds. Monitoring surgical patients in the operating room. Springfield, Ill, Thomas: 197-212

Ballast A (1985). [Signalling when and how?] (Dutch) In: Abstracts Themadag "Ontwikkelingen in de patienten bewaking" 7 Sept. Leiden, Dept Anesthesiology, Univ Hosp Leiden: 25-27

Bauer D, Cavonius CR (1980). Improving the legibility of visual display units through contrast reversal. In: Grandjean E, Vigliani E eds. Ergonomic aspects of visual display terminals. London, Taylor and Francis: 137-142

Bauer D, Bonacker M, Cavonius CR (1981). Influence of VDU screen brightness on the visibility of reflected images. Disp Technol and Appl 2: 242-244

Bauer D, Bonacker M, Cavonius CR (1983). Frame repetition rate for flicker-free viewing of bright VDU screens. Disp Technol and Appl 4: 31-33

Beaumont JO (19??). Computers in intensive care of critically ill patients. 187-193

Beecher HK (1940). The first anesthesia records (Codman, Cushing). Surg Gynecol and Obstet 71: 689-693

Beecher HK, Todd DP (1954). A study of the deaths associated with anesthesia and surgery. Ann Surg 140: 2-34

Beer RHM de (1984). [Monitoring the quality of invasive blood pressure measurements] (Dutch). MSc Thesis, Eindhoven University of Technology, division EME.

Beneken JEW, Blom JA (1983). An integrative patient monitoring approach. In: Gravenstein JS, Newbower RS, Ream AK, Smith NT eds. An integrated approach to monitoring. Boston, Butterworth: 121-131

Beneken JEW, Blom JA, Meijler AP, Cluitmans P, Spierdijk J, Nandorff A, Nijhuis R, Kessel HM van (1983). Computerized data acquisition and display in anesthesia. In: Prakash O, Meij SH, Patterson RW eds. Developments in critical care medicine and anesthesiology. Boston, Nijhoff: 25-43

Beneken JEW, Cluitmans P, Nandorff A, Meijler AP (1983). Automated record keeping. In: Proc 4th Space age monitoring conf. St. Moritz, Switzerland.

Beneken JEW, Gravenstein JS (1986?). Sophisticated alarms in patient monitoring, a methodology based upon systems engineering concepts. In: Gravenstein JS, Newbower RS, Ream AK, Smith NT eds. The anesthesia record and alarms. Boston, Butterworth (In press).

Beneken JEW, Sluijter ME, Blom JA (1974). Computer models of halothane anesthesia; Application leading to servoanesthesia. In: Feldman SA, Leigh JM, Spierdijk J eds. Measurement in Anaesthesia. Leiden University Press, Boerhaave Series 9: 183-200

Berger JJ, Donchin M, Morgan LS, Aa J van der, Gravenstein JS (1984). Perioperative changes in blood pressure and heart rate. Anesth Analg 63: 647-652

Block FE Jr, Burton LW, Rafal MD, Burton K, Newey C, Dowell L, Klein FF, Davis DA, Harmel MH (1985). Two computer-based anesthetic monitors: the Duke automatic monitoring equipment (DAME) system and the MICRODAME. J Clin Monit 1: 30-51

Blom JA, Aa J van der, Jorritsma FF, Beneken JEW, Nandorff A, Spierdijk J , Bijnen A van (1981). A research oriented microcomputer based patient monitoring system. Biomed Tech 26: 135-140

Blom JA, Beneken JEW, Jorritsma FF, Gieles JPM, Nandorff A, Spierdijk J (1981). Erkennung von Trends und Fehlern bei Signalen von Patienten unter Narkose. In: Epple et al. eds. Rechnergestützte Intensivpflege, Schriftenreihe Intensivmedizin, Notfallmedizin, Anasthesiologie, Band 26. Stuttgart, Thieme: 126-130

Blom JA, de Ruyter JAF, Saranummi N, Beneken JEW (1985). Detection of trends in monitored variables. In: Carson ER, Cramp DG, eds. Computers and control in clinical medicine. New York, Plenum: 153-174

Boquet G, Bushman JA, Davenport HT (1980). The anaesthetic machine, a study of function and design. Br J Anaesth 52: 61-67

Bradshaw EG, Thompson GR (1975). Computers in anesthesiology and intensive care. Acta Anaesthesiol Belg Suppl 26: 191-199

Branton P, Oborne DJ (1980). A behavioural study of anaesthetists at work. In: Oborne DJ, Gruneberg MM, Eiser JR eds. Research in psychology and medicine. Vol 1: Physical aspects: pain, stress, diagnosis and organic damage. London, Academic Press: 434-441

Bräuninger U (1983). Lichttechnische Eigenschaften der Bildschirmgeräte aus ergonomischer Sicht. PhD Thesis, Eidgenössische Technische Hochschule, Zürich.

Bruce M, Foster JJ (1982). The visibility of colored characters on colored backgrounds in viewdata displays. Visible Lang 16: 382-390

Buurman R den (1977). [Legibility and comprehensiveness of VDU information] (Dutch). In: Conferentie Beeldschermergonomie, Nederlandse Vereniging voor Ergonomie.

Buys S van den (1985) [Guidelines for the use of CRT displays in the OR] (Dutch). Practical Work Report, Eindhoven University of Technology, division EME.

Cluitmans PJM (1983). [Automation of record-keeping in anesthesia] (Dutch). MSc Thesis, Eindhoven University of technology, division EME.

Colin I (1983). Erkennbarkeit alphanumerischer Symbole auf Datensichtgeräten bei unterschiedlichen Farbkontrasten. Z Arbeitswiss 37: 113-115

Collins JC, Higgins SB, Harris TR, Arnold TG (1981). Patientmonitoring systems: criteria for evaluation and selection. J Clin Eng 6: 111-115

Collins VJ (1960). Fatalities in anesthesia and surgery, fundamental considerations. J Am Med Assoc 172: 549-555

Collins VJ (1976). Records, mortality and medical legal considerations. In: Principles of Anesthesiology 2nd ed. Philadelphia, Lea and Febiger: 31-42

Comroe Jr JH (1978). Retrospectroscope: insights into medical discovery. Menlo Park Cal, Von Gehr.

Comroe Jr JH, Dripps RD (1976). Scientific basis for the support of biomedical science. Science 192: 105-111

Coolegem KG (1984). [Intelligent alarms in a Data Acquisition and Display System] (Dutch). MSc Thesis, Eindhoven University of Technology, division EME.

Coolen J (1985). [Improvements in man-machine-interaction in a patient monitoring system: data entry, data-presentation and lay-out] (Dutch). MSc Thesis, Eindhoven University of Technology, division EME.

Cooper JB, Newbower RS (1975). The anesthesia machine- an accident waiting to happen. In: Psychomotor performance and equipment design: 345-358

Cooper JB, Newbower RS, Kitz RJ (1984). An analysis of major errors and equipment failures in anesthesia management: considerations for prevention and detection. Anesthesiology 60: 34-42

Cooper JB, Newbower RS, Long CD (1979). Applications of the critical-incident technique to the study of anesthesia errors. In: Wollman H et al. eds. Health care delivery in anesthesia. Philadelphia, Stickley

Cooper JB, Newbower RS, Long CD, Mc Peek B (1978). Preventable anesthesia mishaps: a study of human factors. Anesthesiology 49: 399-406

Cooper JB, Newbower RS, Moore JW, Trautman ED (1978). A new anesthesia delivery system. Anesthesiology 49: 310-318

Craig J, Wilson ME (1981). A survey of anaesthetic misadventures. Anaesthesia 36: 933-936

Crul JF, Payne JP (1970). The choice of parameters. In: Crul JF, Payne JP eds. Patient monitoring. Amsterdam, Excerpta Medica: 14-21

Cushing H (1903). On routine determinations of arterial tension in operating room and clinic. Boston Med and Surg J 148: 250-256

Damman P (1985). [The program REPORT] (Dutch). Report Eindhoven University of Technology, division EME.

Davies JM, Strunin L (1984). Anesthesia in 1984: how safe is it? Can Med Assoc J 131: 437-441

Demeester M (1982). Chronicler: Systeme versatile de collecte automatique de memorisation et de monitoring de donnees physiologiques et de donnees cliniques.

Döring B (1976a). Analytical methods in man-machine system development. In: Kraiss KF, Moraal J eds. Introduction to human engineering. Köln, TÜV Rheinland: 293-350

Döring B (1976b). Application of system human engineering. In: Kraiss KF, Moraal J eds. Introduction to human engineering. Köln, TÜV Rheinland: 384-415

Dorsthorst M te (1982). [Design of a graphic display for a Data Acquisition and Display System] (Dutch). MSc Thesis, Eindhoven University of Technology, division EME.

Downing DM (1983). Automated anesthesia record-keeping: measuring fluid administration. Anesthesiology 59: A167

Drenth PJD (1976). Selection and training. In: Kraiss KF, Moraal J eds. Introduction to human engineering. Köln, TÜV Rheinland: 258-292

Dreyfuss H (1967). The measure of man: human factors in design 2nd ed. New York, Whitney Library of Design.

Dripps RD, Eckenhof JE, Vandam LD (1982). Introduction to anesthesia, the principles of safe practice. Philadelphia, Saunders

Drui AB, Behm RJ, Martin WE (1973). Predesign investigation of the anesthesia operational environment. Anesth and Analg 52: 584-591

Duberman SM, Bendixen HH (1984). Concepts of fail-safe in anesthetic practice. Int Anesthesiol Clin 22: 149-165

ECRI (1985). Deaths during general anesthesia: Technology-related, due to human error, or unavoidable? Technology for Anesthesia 5 no 9: 1-11

Farrow SC, Fowkers FGR, Lunn JN, Robertson IB, Sweetnam P (1984). Epidemiology in anaesthesia: a method for predicting hospital mortality. Eur J Anaesthesiol 1: 77-84

Flanagan JC (1954). The critical-incident technique. Psychol Bull 51: 327-358

Fogdall RP (1982). The Post-bypass period. In: Ream AK, Fogdall RP eds. Acute Cardiovascular Management, anesthesia and intensive care. Philadelphia, Lippincott: 456-480

Footerman DS (1983). The use of a whistle discriminator. Anesthesia 38: 672-673

Frazier WT, Paulsen AW, Harbort RA, Odom SH, Haygood WF (1981). Integrated anesthesia delivery/monitoring system with computer assisted anesthetic record generation. In: Proc 55th Congr of the International Anesthesia Research Society, Atlanta, Georgia.

Freiman JA, Chalmers TC, Smith H Jr, Kuebler RR (1978). The importance of beta, the type 2 error and sample size in the design and interpretation of the randomized control trial (Survey of 71 "negative" trials). New Engl J Med 299: 690-694

Galer IAR, Yap BL (1980). Ergonomics in intensive care: Applying human factors data to the design and evaluation of patient monitoring systems. Ergonomics 23: 763-779

Gerbode F (1973). Computerized monitoring of seriously ill patients. J Thorac Cardiovasc Surg 66: 167-174

Gerson GR ed (1981). Monitoring during anesthesia. Boston, Little Brown and Comp: 141

Gezondheidsraad (1978). Advies inzake anesthesiologie. Deel 1: Recente ontwikkelingen in de anesthesiologie. Uitgebracht door een commissie van de Gezondheidsraad aan de Minister en de Staatssecretaris van Volksgezondheid en Milieuhygiëne. Verslagen-adviezen-rapporten no 20.

Gibbon jr JH (1954). Application of a mechanical heart and lung apparatus to cardiac surgery. Minn Med 37: 171-185

Gieles JPM (1978). The automatic detection of disturbances in physiological signals, measured during anaesthesia. MSc Thesis, Eindhoven University of Technology, division EME.

Glaeser DH, Trost RF, Brown DB, Kyle AC, Lenahan MS, Walker CK, Wilson CS, DeBakey ME (1975). A hierarchical minicomputer system for continuous post surgical monitoring. Comput Biomed Res 8: 336-361

Gordh TH, Mostert JW (1978). Anesthetic accidents: case studies. Int Anesthesiol Clin 16

Graafmans J (1986). Working conditions in the operating theatre. Reprint 4th Mediterrenean Conference on Medical and Biological Engineering, Sevilla, Spain. Available from: Project-office for Biomedical and Health-care Technology, Technical University Eindhoven.

Gravenstein JS (1980). Failure to monitor. In: Gravenstein JS, Newbower RS, Ream AK, Smith NT, Barden J eds. Essential noninvasive monitoring in anesthesia. New York, Grune and Stratton: 305-310

Gravenstein JS, Paulus DA (1982). Monitoring practice in clinical anesthesia. Philadelphia, Lippincott

Gravenstein JS, Paulus DA (1986). A semi-automatic anesthesia record. Int J Clin Monit and Comput 2: 251

Gravenstein JS, Steinhaus JE, Volpitto PP (1970). Analysis of manpower in anesthesiology. Anesthesiology 33 no 3: 350-357

Greenburg AG, McClure DK, Fink RM, Goldberg M (1975). Evaluation of a computerized intensive care monitoring system: an application of information utilisation monitoring. In: Martin JA ed. Proc 14th San Diego Biomed Symp: 297-302

Hallen B (1973). Computerized anaesthetic record-keeping. Acta Anaesthesiol Scand (Suppl) 52

Harrison GG (1978). Death attributable to anaesthesia, a 10-year survey (1967-1976). Br J Anaesth 50: 1041-1046

Harrison PB, Ludwig D (1983). Drug interactions on a microcomputer. In: Lindberg DAB, Van Brunt EE, Jenkin MA eds. In: Proc 2nd Congress on Medical Informatics, American Association for Medical Systems and Informatics: 479-483

Hartung HJ, Bender HJ, Osswald PM, Lutz H, Olsson SG (1983). Entwicklung und Einsatz eines computergestützt erstellten Anaesthesieprotokolls. Anaesthesist 32: 205-213

Hees KJJM (1983). [System generated manual and processing of manual entries in a Data Acquisition an Display System] (Dutch). MSc Thesis, Eindhoven University of Technology, division EME.

Heesbeen MThH (1984). [Speed-enhancement in command-interpretation and, computation of hemodynamic parameters in a Data Acquisation and Display System] (Dutch). MSc Thesis, Eindhoven University of Technology, division EME.

Hengst J, Kramer B (1980). [Design of a data acquisition system for patient monitoring during anesthesia] (Dutch). MSc Thesis, Eindhoven University of Technology, division EME.

Hilberman M, Kamm B, Tarter M, Osborn JJ (1975). An evaluation of computer-based patient monitoring at pacific medical center. Comput and Biomed Res 8: 447-460

Hollander M, Wolfe DA (1973). Nonparametric statistical methods. New York, Wiley: 26-33, 115-119

Hollnagel E, Hunt G, Marshall E (1983). The experimental validation of the critical function monitoring system. Preliminary results of analysis. Halden, Norway: OECD Halden Reactor Project. HWR-111

Hovi-Viander M (1980). Death associated with anaesthesia in Finland. Br J Anesth 52: 483-489

Hsiao HS, Tommerdahl MA, Wilcox BR (1983). A color graphics monitor for the operating room. In: Lindberg DAB, Van Brunt EE, Jenkin MA eds. In: Proc 2nd Congress on Medical Informatics, American Association for Medical Systems and Informatics: 233-234

Johanson DC, Edey MA (1981). Lucy: the beginnings of humankind. New York, Simon and Schuster: 231

Jorritsma FF, Gieles JPM, Blom JA, Beneken JEW, Nandorff A, van Bijnen A, Spierdijk J (1979). Error detection in patient monitoring. In: Biomedizinische Technik. Berlin, Schiele und Schon. Ergänzungsband 24: 50-51

Kaplan JA (1983). Development of thoracic anesthesia. In: Kaplan JA ed. Thoracic anesthesia. New York, Churchill Livingstone: 3-8

Karliczek GF, Geus F de, Wiersma G, Oosterhaven S (1985). [Automated data registering during anesthesia] (Dutch). In: Proc Microsymposium NVA: Nieuwe trends in de bewaking tijdens anesthesie 5 Oct Amsterdam.

Kasuga H (1982). An approach for designing a friendly and flexible user interface for an office workstation. In: Proc 7th Int Zurich Seminar on Digital Communications: Man-machine interaction. Inst für Fermeldetechnik, ETH Zürich Switserland: 243-245

Keats AS (1979). What do we know about anesthetic mortality? Anesthesiology 50: 387-392

Keats AS, Siker ES (1985). International symposium on preventable anesthetic morbidity and mortality. Anesthesiology 63: 349-350

Kennedy PJ, Feingold A, Wiener EL, Hosek RS (1976). Analysis of tasks and human factors in anesthesia for coronary-artery bypass. Anesth and Analg current researches 55: 374-377

Kessel HM van (1981). [Development of a Data Acquisition and Display System for patient monitoring during anesthesia] (Dutch). MSc Thesis, Eindhoven University of Technology, division EME.

Kessel HM van, Meijler AP, Hennis PJ, Cluitmans PJM (1987). Comparison between a handwritten and automated anesthesia record. In: Gravenstein JS, Newbower RS, Ream AK, Smith NT eds. The automated anesthesia record and alarms. Boston, Butterworth (In press).

Klövekorn WP, Richter J, Mendler N, Sebening F (1976). Computer assisted intensive care monitoring. In: Proc. 3rd Conf Computers in cardiology. New York, IEEE: 237-241

Kragt H (1982). Process-alarm systems. In: Edman TR, Bergman H, eds. European Research in Process Control: Human interactions with computer based systems.

Krischer JP (1982). Outcome criteria for evaluating anesthesia care. In: Grundy BL, Gravenstein JS eds. The quality of care in anesthesia. Springfield Ill, Thomas: 141-151

Laird-Meeter K (1983). Results of ten years aorto-coronary bypass surgery at the thoraxcenter, Rotterdam. PhD Thesis, Erasmus University of Rotterdam.

Lange de JJ (1985). [Monitoring in anesthesia, present and future] (Dutch). Tijdschr Tech Gezondheidszorg no 2: 44-45

Lavoir RGEMR van de (1983). [Development of an off-line display editor for a Data Acquisition and Display System] (Dutch). MSc Thesis, Eindhoven University of Technology, division EME.

Lee JA, Atkinson RS (1973). A synopsis of anesthesia. 7th ed. Bristol, John Wright: 1-25

Leebeek HJ (1980). Met het oog op beeldschermen. Instituut voor Zintuig Fysiologie, 12F No20.

Lewis FJ, Deller S, Quinn M, Lee B, Will R, Raines J (1972). Continuous patient monitoring with a small digital computer. Comput and Biomed Res 5: 411-428

Lunn JN, Mushin WW (1982). Mortality associated with anaesthesia. London, Nuffield Provincial Hospitals Trust.

Manteleers JJH (1985). [Critical incidents during anesthesia] (Dutch). Report Practical Work, Eindhoven University of Technology, division EME.

Marx GF, Mateo CV, Orkin LR (1973). Computer analysis of postanesthetic deaths. Anesthesiology 39: 54-58

McClure DK, Greenburg AG, Fink RM (1975). Computerized patient monitoring- a critical evaluation. In: Martin JA ed. Proc 14th San Diego Biomed Symp 14: 289-295

McCormick EJ, Sanders MS (1983). Human factors in engineering and design. 5th ed. New York, McGraw-Hill.

McEwen JA, Jenkins LC (1983). Complications of and improvements to breathing circuit monitors for anesthesia ventilators. Med Instrum 17: 70-74

Meijler AP, Beneken JEW (1987). Data Acquisition and Display: A system with centralized display, automatic record keeping and intelligent alarms. In: Gravenstein JS, Newbower RS, Ream AK, Smith NT eds. The automated anesthesia record and alarms. Boston, Butterworth (In press).

Meijler AP, Beneken JEW, Nandorff A, van Kessel HM, Spierdijk J (1983). A data acquisition and display system for improved medical pattern recognition. In: Beneken JEW, Lavelle SM eds. Lecture notes in medical informatics Vol 22. Objective medical decision-making; systems approach in acute disease. Berlin, Springer: 101-112

Meijler AP, Blom J, Kessel H van, Beneken J, Spierdijk J, Nandorff A, Nijhuis R (1982). On a flexible system for patient monitoring during anesthesia. In: Proc World Congress on Medical Physics and Biomedical Engineering. Hamburg: A9.08

Meijler FL, Robles de Medina EO, Zimmerman ANE (1975). Electrocardiography for intensive-care units. Amsterdam, Excerpta Medica.

Mikolajczuk A (1974). Three years of experience with computer-assisted patient monitoring. In: Anderson J, Forsythe JM eds. Proc 1st World Conf on Medical Informatics Vol 2. Amsterdam, North-Holland: 787-794

Mitchell MM, Meathe EA, Ozaki GT, Saidman LJ (1979). Application of computer technology to intraoperative patient monitoring. Anesthesiology 51: S334

Mitchell RR, Feihl F, Osborn JJ (1983). A clinical evaluation of a knowledge based respiratory alarm system.

Moraal J (1976). What is human engineering? In: Kraiss KF, Moraal J eds. Introduction to human engineering. Köln, TÜV Rheinland: 1-27

Murch GM (1984). Physiological Principles for the effective use of color. IEEE Comput Graphics and Appl 4 no 11: 49-54

Murray G (1981) ed. User-friendly systems. Infotech State of the Art Report, Series 9 no 4. Maidenhead Berksh, Pergamon Infotech.

Mushin WW, Rendell-Baker L, Morton HJV et al. (1953). Discussion: are anaesthetic records worth keeping? Proc R Soc Med 46: 739-746

Nandorff A, Spierdijk Joh, Beneken J, Blom J, Jorritsma F, Bijnen A van, Bruyn N de (1980). Trends in patient monitoring during surgery. Abstract 7th World congress of Anesthesiologists, Hamburg: 242

Nes FL van (1983). New characters for teletext with improved legibility. In: Annual Progress Report 1983. Eindhoven, IPO: 108-113

Newbower RS, Cooper JB, Edmondson JE, Maier WR (1981 a). Graphics-tablet for data entry in computer-assisted anesthesia record-keeping. In: Hefferman HG ed. Proc 5th Annual Symp on Computer Applications in Medical Care Washington DC: 139-142

Newbower RS, Cooper JB, Long CD (1981 b). Learning from anesthesia mishaps. Quality Rev Bull: 10-16

New South Wales (1970). Special Committee Investigating Deaths under Anaesthesia: Report on 745 classified cases, 1960-1968. [R Holland secretary] Med J Aust 1: 573-594

Noback (1983). Intraoperative monitoring. In: Kaplan JA ed. Thoracic anesthesia. New York, Churchill Livingstone: 197-246

Noel TA (1986). Computerized anesthesia records may be dangerous. Anesthesiology 64: 300

Oborne DJ (1985). Computers at work- A behavioural approach. Chichester, Wiley.

Ornato JP, Fennigkoh L, Jaeger C (1981). The electronic clipboard: an automated system for accurately recording events during a cardiac arrest. Ann Emerg Med 10: 138-141

Pace NL (1985). But what does monitoring do to patient outcome? Int J Clin Mon and Comp 1: 197-200

Paget NS, Lambert TF, Sridhar K (1981). Factors affecting an anaesthetist's work: some findings on vigilance and performance. Anaesth and Intensive Care 9: 359-365

Pearlman AL, Gurman GM (1985). Toward a unified monitoring system during anesthesia. Int J Clin Monit and Comput 2: 21-27

Peters RM (1979). Monitoring of ventilation in the anesthetized patient. In: Gravenstein JS, Newbower RS, Ream AK, Smith NT, Barden JD eds. Monitoring surgical patients in the operating room. Springfield Ill, Thomas: 142-149

Peters RM, Knight MK, Brimm JE, Hogan JS, Shelton R (1985). A personal computer system for testing gas exchange, heart, lungs, ventilator, pump. Int J Clin Monit and Comp 2: 113-119

Phillips OC, Capizzi LS (1974). Anesthesia mortality. In: Safar P ed. Public health aspects of critical care medicine and anesthesiology. Philadelphia, Davis: 220-244

Pierce EC Jr (1984). Historical perspectives (analysis of anesthetic mishaps). In: Pierce EC, Cooper JB eds (1984). Analysis of anesthetic mishaps. Int Anesthesiol Clin 22: 1-16

Plasman JLC (1981). An introducion to the analysis of the arterial and venous pressure waves. MSc Thesis, Eindhoven University of Technology, division EME.

Pluth JR, Smith HC, Schultz GL (1972). The computerized intensive-care unit: a comparative evaluation. In: Anesth. and Postop care in cardiac surgery. Section 4, Chapter 24: 152-156

Pogulanik J (1980). Accidental disconnection of anaesthetic breathing systems. Anaesthesia 35: 825-827

Prakash O, Borden SG van der, Meij SH, Rulf ENR, Hugenholtz PG (1984b). A microcomputer based charting system for documentation of circulatory, respiratory and pharmacological data during anesthesia. Int J Clin Monit and Comput 1: 155-160

Prakash O, Meij SH, Borden SG van der (1984a). On-line monitoring of hemodynamic and respiratory parameters in the operating theatre and the ICU. Int Care world 1: 36-43

Pütsep E (1979). Modern hospital international planning practices. London, Lloyd-Luke: 223-230

Radl GW, Experimental investigations for optimal presentationmode and colours of symbols on the CRT-screen. In: Grandjean E, Vigliani E eds. Ergonomic aspects of visual display terminals. London, Taylor and Francis: 127-135

Raison JCA, Beaumont JO, Russell JAG, Osborn JJ, Gerbode F (1968). Alarms in an intensive care unit: an interim compromise. Comput Biomed Res 1: 556-564

Rampil IJ, Flemming DC (1978). An inexpensive microcomputer trend monitoring system. In: Jaron D ed. Proc 6th New England Bioeng Conf. Oxford, Pergamon: 67-70

Ream AK (1982). Monitoring concepts and techniques. In: Ream AK, Fogdall RP eds. Acute Cardiovascular Management: anesthesia and intensive care. Philadelphia, Lippincott : 139-160

Ream AK (1982). Cardiopulmonary Bypass. In: Ream AK, Fogdall RP eds. Acute Cardiovascular Management, anesthesia and intensive care. Philadelphia, Lippincott: 420-455

Rendell-Baker L (1982). Problems with anesthetic gas machines and their solutions. Int Anesthesiol Clin 20: 1-82

Rijswijk EAHM van (1986). [An estimation-algorithm for measuring and improving the quality of invasive blood pressure measurements] (Dutch). MSc Thesis Eindhoven University of Technology, division EME.

Robicsek F, Masters ThN, Reichertz PL, Daugherty HK, Cook JW (1977). Three years experience with computer-based intensive care of patients following open heart and major vascular surgery. Surgery 81: 12-21.

Roo J de (1980). [Investigation and design of anesthesia and monitoring equipment] (Dutch). MSc Thesis, Delft University of Technology, Dept Industrial Engineering.

Saidman LJ, Smith NT eds (1984). Monitoring in anesthesia 2nd edition. Boston, Butterworth.

Sanders AF (1976). Experimental methods in Human Engineering In: Kraiss KF, Moraal J eds. Introduction to human engineering. Köln, TÜV Rheinland: 351-383

Sarnat AJ (1983). Computerized speech recognition for anesthesia record keeping. Med Instrum 17: 25-27

Sarnat AJ, Quinn ML, Smith NT (1981). A preliminary evaluation of computerized speech recognition for anesthesia. Anesthesiology 55: A128

Schillings H, Scharnberg B, Sabean RM, Ehlers CT (1978). Ein neues Konzept computerunterstützter Schwerkrankenüberwachung: Göttinger Informationssystem für Intensivpflege (GISI). Methods Inf Med 17: 173-176

Schneider AJL (1982). The validity of data from anesthesia records. In: Grundy BL, Gravenstein JS eds. The quality of care in anesthesia. Springfield Ill, Thomas: 100-113

Schneider AJL, Knoke JD, Zollinger RM, McLaren CE, Baetz WR (1979). Morbidity prediction using pre- and intraoperative data. Anesthesiology 51: 4-10

Schoor BFW (1986). [The trenddetection algorithm as a basis for an expert system for intelligent alarms] (Dutch). MSc Thesis ,Eindhoven University of Technology, division EME.

Seed RF, Welsh EA (1976). Anaesthetic records in Great Britain and Ireland. Anaesthesia 31: 1199-1210

Sheppard LC, Kouchoukos NT (1976). Computers as monitors. Anesthesiology 45: 250-259

Sheppard LC, Kouchoukos NT, Shotts JF, Wallace FD (1975). Regulation of mean arterial pressure by computer control of vasoactive agents in postoperative patients. In: Proc 2nd Conf Computers in Cardiology. New York IEEE: 91-94

Shubin H, Weil MH, Palley N, Afifi AA (1971). Monitoring the critically ill patient with the aid of a digital computer. Comput and Biomed Res 4: 460-473

Simons AJR, Pronk RAF (1983). Automatic EEG monitoring during anesthesia. In: Prakash O, Meij SH, Patterson RW eds. Developments in critical care medicine and anesthesiology. Boston, Nijhoff: 227-257

Sisson N, Parkinson S, Snowbe K (1983). Design methodology for menu structures. In: Proc Ann Conf on computers and communications. Los Angeles IEEE: 557-560

Smalhout B (1972). De dood op tafel. Inaugurele rede. Utrecht, Oosthoek.

Smalhout B, Kalenda Z (1975). An atlas of capnography Vol 1. Zeist, Kerckebosch.

Smith NT (1983). Machines versus people. In: Proc 4th Space Age Monitoring Conf. St. Moritz, Switzerland.

Snow J (1958). On Chloroform and other anaesthetics: Their action and administration. London, Churchill.

Sodal IE, Swanson GD (1980). Mass spectrometer in patient monitoring. In: Gravenstein JS, Newbower RS, Ream AK, Smith NT, Barden J eds. Essential noninvasive monitoring in anesthesia. New York, Grune and Stratton: 217-234

Spierdijk J, Nandorff A (1974). The difference between measurement and monitoring: what is worth measuring? In: Feldman SA, Leigh JM, Spierdijk J eds. Measurement in anesthesia. Leiden University Press, Boerhaave series no 9: 3-12

Spooner RB, Kirby RR (1984). Equipment-related anesthetic incidents. Int Anesthesiol Clin 22: 133-147

Stap RAM van der (1982). [An inventarisation of techniques for the evaluation of a medical electrotechnical apparatus] (Dutch). Practical Work Report, Eindhoven University of Technology, division EME.

Stetz CW, Miller RG, Kelly GE, Raffin TA (1982). Reliability of the thermodilution method in the determination of cardiac output in clinical practice. Am Rev Respir Dis 126: 1001-1004

Swoboda A, Polonius MJ, Schaldach M, Rodewald G (1976). Rechnerunterstützte postoperative Intensivmedizin der Herz- und Gefäßchirurgie. In: Schneider B und Schönenberger R eds. Datenverarbeitung im Gesundheitswesen. Berlin, Springer: 35-41

Toffler A (1981). The third wave. Toronto, Bantam books: 140

Trispel S, Klocke H, Rau G (1981). Aspekte der Interaktion mit einem Anasthesie-Monitoring-System. Aachen, Forschungsbericht Helmholtz Institut: 64-67

Trispel S, Klocke H, Rau G (1985). Verfahren und Techniken zur Überwachung und Protokollierung des Narkoseverlaufs. Aachen, Forschungsbericht Helmoholtz Institut: 27-38

Trispel S, Rau G (1982). User guidance strategies for the visual interface with virtual control elements. In: Proc 7th Int Zürich Seminar on Digital Communications: Man-machine interaction. Institut für Fernmeldtechnik der ETH Zürich: 247-252

Utting JE, Gray TC, Shelley FC (1979). Human misadventure in anaesthesia. Can Anaesth Soc J 26: 472-478

Vorst JHM van der (1985). [A multi-microprocessorsystem as a front-end processor in the Data Acquisition and Display System] (Dutch). MSc Thesis, Eindhoven University of Technology, division EME.

Warner HR (1969). Computer-based patient monitoring. In: Stacy RW and Waxmann BD eds. Computers in Biomedical research 3. New York, Academic Press: 239-251

Warner DL, Essin DJ, Steen SN (1985). Paediatric anaesthetic management with the aid of a computer. Int J Clin Monit and Comput 2: 9-14

Websters (1979). New Collegiate Dictionary. Springfield Mass, Merriam.

Werf T van der (1965). [Direct and indirect measurement of blood flow. On the possibilities of thermistor catheters] (Dutch). PhD thesis, Rijks Universiteit Groningen.

Westenskow DR, Jordan WS, Hayes JK, East TD (1983). Computer control of anesthesia delivery. In: Proc 2nd Congr Comp in Anesth and Int Care. Boston, Nijhoff: 269-278

Whitesell R, Asiddao C, Jablonski J. (priv. comm.) Comparison of the accuracy of computerized and conventionally recorded anesthesia records.

Wiener F, Weil MH (1978). Computer based monitoring and data management in critical care. Methods Inf Med 17: 252-260

Wood EH (1978). Evolution of instrumentation and techniques for study of cardiovascular dynamics from the Thirties to 1980, Alza Lecture. Ann Biomed Eng 6: 250-309

Yelderman M, New W Jr, Rosenthal M, Ream AK (1980). Improved clinical measurement of pulmonary vascular resistance. Anesthesiology 52: 365-369

Zandbergen PCL (1986). [The conversion of patient files to a relational database] (Dutch). MSc Thesis Eindhoven University of Technology, division EME.
Zegers-de Beyl R (1985). [Towards an integrated workstation] (Dutch) In: Abstracts Themadag "Ontwikkelingen in de patienten bewaking" 7 Sept. Leiden, Dept Anesthesiology, Univ Hosp Leiden: 25-27
Zelders T (1986). [The price of more safety in anesthesia] (Dutch) Med Cont 41 no 9: 267-270
Zollinger RM, Kreul JF, Schneider AJL (1977). Man-made versus computer-generated anesthesia records. J Surg Res 22: 419-424

Subject Index

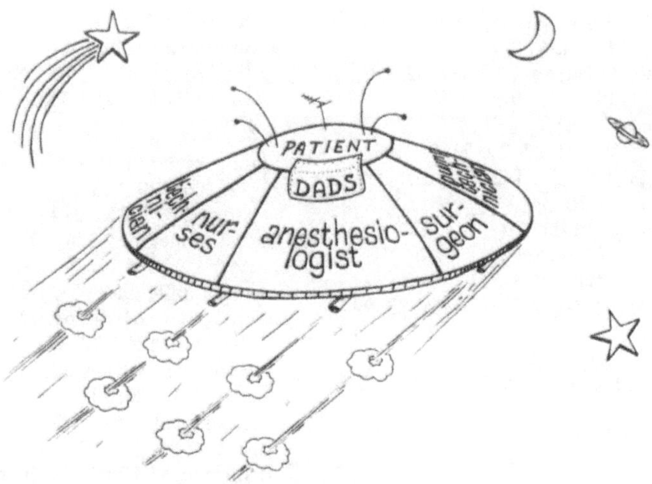
PATIENT
DADS
tech-
ni-
cian
nur-
ses
anesthesio-
logist
sur-
geon